100 Questions & Answers About Triple Negative Breast Cancer

Carey K. Anders, MD

Assistant Professor
Lineberger Comprehensive Cancer Center
University of North Carolina
Chapel Hill, NC

Nancy U. Lin, MD

Assistant Professor of Medicine
Dana-Farber Cancer Institute
Boston, MA

JONES & BARTLETT
L E A R N I N G

World Headquarters
Jones & Bartlett Learning
5 Wall Street
Burlington, MA 01803
978-443-5000
info@jblearning.com
www.jblearning.com

Jones & Bartlett Learning
Canada
6339 Ormindale Way
Mississauga, Ontario L5V 1J2
Canada

Jones & Bartlett Learning
International
Barb House, Barb Mews
London W6 7PA
United Kingdom

Jones & Bartlett Learning books and products are available through most bookstores and online booksellers. To contact Jones & Bartlett Learning directly, call 800-832-0034, fax 978-443-8000, or visit our website, www.jblearning.com.

Substantial discounts on bulk quantities of Jones & Bartlett Learning publications are available to corporations, professional associations, and other qualified organizations. For details and specific discount information, contact the special sales department at Jones & Bartlett Learning via the above contact information or send an email to specialsales@jblearning.com.

Production Credits
Executive Publisher: Christopher Davis
Special Projects Editor: Kathy Richardson
Associate Editor: Laura Burns
Production Editor: Leah Corrigan
Associate Marketing Manager: Katie Hennessy
Manufacturing and Inventory Control Supervisor: Amy Bacus
Composition: Cenveo Publisher Services
Cover Design: Carolyn Downer
Cover Images: (top left) © Andresr/ShutterStock, Inc., (top right) © Juriah Mosin/ShutterStock, Inc., (bottom) © Monkey Business Images/Dreamstime.com
Printing and Binding: Malloy, Inc.
Cover Printing: Malloy, Inc.

Library of Congress Cataloging-in-Publication Data
Anders, Carey K.
  100 questions and answers about triple negative breast cancer/Carey K. Anders and Nancy U. Lin.
    p. cm.
  Includes bibliographical references and index.
  ISBN 978-1-4496-0930-6 (pbk. : alk. paper)
  1. Breast—Cancer—Miscellanea. 2. Breast—Cancer—Popular works. I. Lin, Nancy U.
II. Title. III. Title: One hundred questions and answers about triple negative breast cancer.
  RC280.B8A4943 2012
  616.99'449—dc22
                          2010047561

6048

Printed in the United States of America
15 14 13 12 11   10 9 8 7 6 5 4 3 2 1

Contents

Contents

When I first found out my cancer was triple negative, I thought it meant I did not have to take any extra medications. I thought that was a good thing. It was caught early stage 1. That also meant no chemo, I would have my mastectomy and I would be cured and I would move on with my life. I then got the earth shattering news that I was BRCA1+. I had no family history, how could this be? This is when I hit the net and began my research. It was on the TNBCF site where I got a real education on the true nature of triple negative disease. It was as if I was punched in the stomach. The old saying "early detection, early cure" did not apply to me. Being triple negative means there is no specific targeted or hormonal treatment out there for me. Being triple negative means I am at a higher risk for recurrence, regardless of diagnostic stage. Being triple negative means I am at a higher risk of distant metastases.

Today I am more than two years out from diagnosis. I have had several additional risk reducing surgeries. I have learned to embrace my new normal. This does not mean I live without fear on a daily basis; however, the fear does not own me. I am cancer free. Today I live my life to the fullest, grateful for that gift. In turn I wish to share my gift by being there to assist anyone who needs an ear, a voice, a shoulder, or a hug. I also am very hopeful that the day will come when there will be personalized cancer treatment, and all breast cancers will be treated as individual diseases. I am even more hopeful that scientists will have a breakthrough and find a way to prevent breast cancer. They have been uncovering so many genetic factors; they are so close. I want my children to live their lives without fear and wonder of when…

PART ONE

The Basics of Breast Cancer, Specifically Triple Negative Breast Cancer

What is cancer? Specifically, what is breast cancer?

Is it true that breast cancer is the most common cancer among women in the United States? How many breast cancer survivors are living in the United States today?

What does "triple negative" breast cancer mean?

More . . .

1. What is cancer? Specifically, what is breast cancer?

Every organ in the body is made up of various kinds of **cells**, which are easily distinguished from one another in form and function. Brain cells are different from blood cells, which are distinguishable from liver or skin cells, for example. Cells normally divide in an orderly way to produce more cells only when they are needed. Each cell is pre-programmed to have a specific life cycle, and normal cells contain a trigger that begins the process of cell death. This process of regulated growth and death helps keep the body healthy.

Occasionally, cells become abnormal and divide without control or order, or fail to die at the appropriate time. If cells divide when new cells are not needed, they form too much tissue. The mass or lump of extra tissue, called a **tumor**, can be **benign** or **malignant**.

Benign tumors are not cancer. They can usually be removed, and in most cases, they don't come back. Most important, the cells in benign tumors do not invade other tissues and do not spread to other parts of the body. Benign breast tumors are not a threat to life.

Malignant tumors are cancer. Cancer cells that arise from, for instance, breast tissue grow and divide out of control; they also become **undifferentiated**, which means they lose the distinguishing characteristics of the original tissue (i.e., normal breast). They can invade and damage nearby tissues and organs. Also, breast cancer cells can break away from a malignant tumor and enter the bloodstream or lymphatic system. That is how breast cancer spreads and forms secondary tumors in other parts of the body. The spread of cancer is called **metastasis**.

Cells

Basic elements of tissues; the appearance and composition of individual cells are unique to the tissue they compose.

Tumor

A mass or lump of extra tissue; a tumor can be benign or malignant.

Benign

Not cancerous.

Malignant

Cancerous; growing rapidly and out of control.

Undifferentiated

Cells that are not specialized and are somewhat immature.

Metastasis

The spread of cancer to other organs.

2. Is it true that breast cancer is the most common cancer among women in the United States? How many breast cancer survivors are living in the United States today?

According to the American Cancer Society, breast cancer is the most common cancer diagnosed among women in the Unites States. It is estimated that close to 190,000 women living in the United States were diagnosed with invasive breast cancer during the year 2009. Despite advances in current treatments, approximately 40,000 women died from breast cancer during this same year. Only lung cancer accounts for more cancer deaths in women in the United States today.

Although breast cancer is a very frightening and dangerous disease, most women diagnosed with breast cancer are cured completely and go on to live full and happy lives. It is estimated that there are over 2 million breast cancer survivors currently living in the United States.

3. What does "triple negative" breast cancer mean?

Breast cancer is no longer viewed as one disease, but rather a group of diseases under the umbrella of "breast cancer." Different types of breast cancer are defined, in part, by factors that promote breast cancer cell growth. These factors include **receptors** that live on breast cancer cell surfaces and other **genes** that signal for cancer cell growth.

The two receptors most commonly found on the outer surface of breast cancer cells are the **estrogen** and **progesterone** receptors. It is estimated that approximately two-thirds of all breast cancers have estrogen receptors

Receptors

Protein molecules that are embedded in the outside surface of cells; when receptors are activated, cancer cells may be stimulated to grow.

Genes

Sequences of DNA which comprise the genetic material of living organisms.

Estrogen

A female hormone related to child-bearing and the menstrual cycle.

Progesterone

A female hormone involved in the menstrual cycle and child-bearing.

3

and/or progesterone receptors on their surface; thus, in the presence of these female hormones, the abnormal cells are signaled to grow and divide. A third factor, a gene called *HER2/neu*, is frequently amplified in human breast cancers. The *HER2* gene is amplified in approximately one-third of all breast cancers. *HER2* overexpression can also overlap with expression of the estrogen and/or progesterone receptors.

Triple negative breast cancer is a unique subset of breast cancer that lacks all three factors. There is no expression of the estrogen or progesterone receptors, and the *HER2* gene is not amplified. Thus, the term "triple negative." Triple negative breast cancer makes up approximately 20% of all human breast cancers and is characterized by unique biologic characteristics and treatment options.

HER2/neu

A gene which is over-expressed in approximately 20% of breast cancers and can increase its aggressiveness.

Triple negative breast cancer

Breast cancers that lack expression of the estrogen receptor, progesterone receptor, and HER2 protein.

4. Triple negative breast cancer seems rare compared to other types of breast cancer. How many women are diagnosed with triple negative breast cancer worldwide?

It is estimated that close to 1 million women worldwide are diagnosed with breast cancer of any subtype. Of these 1 million women, approximately 175,000 are diagnosed with triple negative breast cancer. Although it may seem rare compared to other types of breast cancers, triple negative breast cancer is the subject of tremendous research. So, although not the most common of all breast cancers, scientists and doctors are making great strides in understanding what makes triple negative breast cancers grow and in developing novel treatments for this disease.

5. If triple negative breast cancer is not reliant on the estrogen and/or progesterone receptors or the HER2 gene, then what makes it grow?

Scientists continue to study triple negative breast cancer to help answer this very question. Although it is not completely understood, there are some characteristics unique to triple negative breast cancer that might explain what drives growth of these abnormal cells. Scientists have shown that approximately two-thirds of triple negative breast cancers express the **epithelial growth factor receptor** (**EGFR**, also known as *HER1*) on their cell surface. This might explain how some triple negative breast cancers grow; a strategy of blocking EGFR has been tested to treat triple negative breast cancer based on this and other findings.

Another gene, called *TP53*, has been found to be mutated in over 80% of triple negative breast cancers. *TP53* is a tumor suppressor gene, thus when it does not function properly (or is mutated), cells grow out of control and form cancers. Loss of *TP53* function may also explain how some triple negative breast cancers grow.

Finally, the gene *BRCA1* is responsible for repairing DNA damage. Cells within our bodies undergo DNA damage every day, and the *BRCA1* gene helps repair this damage. Otherwise, cells may become abnormal, which can lead to cancer. Women who have mutations in their *BRCA1* gene are at high risk of developing breast and **ovarian cancers**. If they develop breast cancer, their cancers are more likely to be triple negative. More detailed discussions on *BRCA* **mutations** will be presented later in this book.

Epithelial growth factor receptor (EGFR, also known as HER1)

A receptor expressed on the surface of many cancer cells; EGFR is frequently over-expressed in triple negative breast cancer.

TP53

A tumor suppressor gene; when abnormal cells can grow uncontrollably and form tumors.

BRCA1

A tumor suppressor gene; certain mutations in this gene lead to an increased risk of breast and ovarian cancers.

Ovarian cancer

Cancer beginning in the ovaries, sometimes genetically related to breast cancer.

BRCA mutations

Mutations in either the BRCA1 or 2 gene that leads to inherited breast cancer.

The Basics of Breast Cancer, Specifically Triple Negative Breast Cancer

PART TWO

Risk Factors and Prevention

What are the risk factors for developing
breast cancer?

Are the risk factors for triple negative breast cancer
the same as for other types of breast cancer?

Is it true that younger women are diagnosed
with triple negative breast cancer?

More . . .

6. What are the risk factors for developing breast cancer?

Certain risk factors that may contribute to the development of breast cancer are more influential than others. We will discuss general risk factors for breast cancer below.

Age

The biggest single risk factor for breast cancer is age, a risk that is always increasing. The average age of women diagnosed with breast cancer is in the early 60s. This does not mean that younger women in their 30s and 40s don't get breast cancer, because they do; it simply means that the older a woman gets, the greater her likelihood of getting breast cancer, taking into account other risk factors.

It is estimated that 1 in 8 women will have breast cancer during her lifetime. While frightening, it is a cumulative statistic, covering a lifetime of over 80 years. More specific statistics that account for a woman's age tell a different (and somewhat more reassuring) story: A woman in her late 30s, for instance, has about a 1 in 257 chance of getting breast cancer, whereas a woman in her mid-50s has about a 1 in 36 chance. Even in women 70 years old, the chance of developing cancer is roughly 1 in 12. So what does this mean? It means as women age, they need to be vigilant about changes in their breasts because their risk for developing breast cancer has increased.

Personal History

Other risk factors include details related to a woman's personal history. Chief among these is a woman's past medical history of breast or ovarian cancer. It is important to note that this risk is not a risk of developing a recurrence or metastasis of any of these cancers; it is a risk of developing an unrelated, new cancer in the unaffected breast. Women who have had breast cancer previously stand a greater chance of having a new cancer develop in their breast tissue.

Breast cancer risk may also be related to the timing of normal physiological processes, such as **menarche** (start of menstruation) and **menopause** (end of menstrual periods). If a woman's menarche occurs prior to the age of 12 years, or if her menopause comes after the age of 55 years, or both, then the time frame during which her body is exposed to higher levels of female hormones (i.e., estrogen and progesterone) is extended, and she stands a slightly greater chance of developing breast cancer. Women who have had no pregnancies, or whose first pregnancy occurred after age 30 years, are at slightly greater risk than women who had a child before this age. Moreover, the decision to breast-feed one's children, as opposed to bottle-feeding, seems to affect breast cancer risk, with **breast-feeding** contributing to decreased cancer rates (the longer a woman breast-feeds, the lower her risk of breast cancer). Radiation exposure at any point in her lifetime, but especially exposure related to treatment of childhood cancer occurring in the chest area, can contribute to a woman's risk of developing breast cancer. Postmenopausal estrogen therapy is associated with increased risk, particularly in those taking a combination of estrogen and progestin, but the majority of recent studies do not confirm such risk from oral contraceptives.

Family History

Many people believe that breast cancer is a disease that runs in families. Statistically speaking, this is not necessarily true; over 90% of women who are diagnosed

Menarche
Start of menstruation.

Menopause
End of menstrual periods.

Breast-feeding
Breast-feeding is the feeding of an infant or young child with breast milk directly from female human breasts.

with breast cancer do not have a specific and/or identified gene mutation that runs in their family that caused their breast cancer. Nevertheless, women with a blood relative who has had breast cancer do have a greater risk, particularly if it's a close relative (mother, sister, or daughter); the specific genetic cause, however, remains unknown.

Women with a significant family history of breast and/or ovarian cancer have an increased risk of getting these cancers through an inherited cause. A significant family history is defined as having two or more close family members who have had breast and/or ovarian cancer, particularly if the breast cancer in the family members has been found before the age of 50 years. A close family member can be your mother, sister, grandparent (on either your mother's or father's side), mother's sister, or father's sister. Your father, brother, or uncle would also be considered close family members if they had breast cancer, but breast cancer is very rare in men. Your family history of cancer can be assessed by a doctor or other healthcare professional trained in genetics who will determine if you have a significant family history of breast and/or ovarian cancer. Having this information may help you learn about your cancer risk and help you decide if you should consider genetic testing for the known cancer genes such as *BRCA1* and **BRCA2**. This subject is discussed in later questions.

BRCA2

A tumor suppressor gene; certain mutations in this gene lead to an increased risk of breast cancer, ovarian cancer, prostate cancer, and male breast cancer.

Diet and Physical Fitness

Research suggests that a person's diet may affect the chances of getting some types of cancer. Women who are overweight or obese, particularly older women as noted previously, also have a greater risk. Steroids in our blood's circulation are converted to estrogen in adipose tissues (i.e., fat cells in the body) via an enzyme called aromatase. Therefore, the more adipose tissue, the higher the amount of circulating estrogen, which may account for this increased risk of breast cancer. Although there are no specific foods shown to increase one's risk of breast cancer, it is recommended that women consume a well-balanced diet (following the U.S. Department of Agriculture's dietary guidelines), rich in fruits and vegetables. Maintaining good physical fitness through exercise has been suggested as a potential way to lower cancer risk. Although there is no direct evidence that exercise itself prevents cancer, exercise reduces estrogen levels, fights obesity, lowers insulin levels, and boosts the immune system, all of which can aid in cancer prevention.

Race

In the United States, whites (especially those of northern European descent) have a higher incidence of breast cancer compared to nonwhites. African American and Hispanic women have the next highest incidence, with the lowest rates overall occurring in Korean, American Indian, and Vietnamese women. However, the incidence in nonwhites, specifically African Americans, is increasing, particularly in women younger than 60 years. In women younger than 40 years, the incidence is higher for African American women than white women, and African American women commonly have the highest overall mortality of all groups. High mortality of African American breast cancer patients may be related to the fact that they often are diagnosed with cancer when they have reached a later stage of the disease, which is more difficult to treat.

Though it was previously thought that the problem was one of public health awareness—that African American women were not being educated in the need for breast self-exams, mammograms, and other early detection strategies—recent studies have shown that a major reason for the disparity in disease progression and mortality is indeed biologic in nature. African American women usually are diagnosed at a younger age than their white counterparts and their tumors often have more aggressive characteristics. For example, triple negative breast cancers are about twice as common in African American women, compared to white women (see Question 9). Early detection, breast cancer awareness, and appropriate treatment can be lifesaving for many women with breast cancer, and this is likely especially the case in African American women.

7. Are the risk factors for triple negative breast cancer the same as for other types of breast cancer?

Given that triple negative breast cancer is a unique subset of breast cancer, researchers sought to determine if risk factors for triple negative breast cancer are the same or different compared to more common types of breast cancer (i.e., estrogen receptor- and/or progesterone receptor-positive and *HER2*-negative breast cancers). Interestingly, in studying large populations of thousands of women with breast cancer, it has become apparent that the risk factors associated with triple negative breast cancer differ when compared to other types of breast cancer. For instance, increases in the risk of triple negative breast cancer were observed with increasing number of live births (**increased parity**) and *younger age at first full-term pregnancy* (<26 years of age). If you recall from our earlier discussion, these risks are somewhat different from the typical risk factors associated with breast cancer across the board.

Increased parity

Having many children.

In addition, researchers showed that women diagnosed with triple negative breast cancer *breast-fed for shorter durations* when compared to women with estrogen receptor- and/or progesterone receptor-positive and *HER2*-negative breast cancer. Interestingly, prior *use of* **lactation suppressants** was associated with increases in the risk of triple negative breast cancer, but not estrogen receptor- and/or progesterone receptor-positive and *HER2*-negative breast cancer. These studies show that the risks for triple negative breast cancer may differ from other more common types of breast cancer; moreover, preventive strategies must be tailored to individual breast cancer subtypes, as a "one-size-fits-all" approach may not be sufficient (or individualized enough) for patients at higher risk for breast cancer.

Lactation suppressants
Medicines that stop breast milk production.

8. Is it true that younger women are diagnosed with triple negative breast cancer?

Large population-based studies evaluating hundreds of women with breast cancer have shown that triple negative breast cancer is more commonly diagnosed in younger, premenopausal women when compared to older, postmenopausal women. This finding does not mean that all young women are at high risk for developing triple negative breast cancer. It may help explain, however, if you are diagnosed with breast cancer at a younger age, why your breast cancer is classified as triple negative.

9. I've read that triple negative breast cancer is more common among African American patients. Is this true?

In addition to the young age link, researchers have shown that triple negative breast cancer is more commonly diagnosed in African American patients when compared to non–African American patients. As mentioned in Question 6, African American women often have poorer breast cancer survival. One explanation is that African American women are often diagnosed with faster-growing, more aggressive forms of breast cancer—triple negative breast cancer—which may account for this difference in outcome.

Moreover, when combining race and age, researchers have shown that younger and premenopausal African American patients who are diagnosed with breast cancer are more commonly diagnosed with triple negative breast cancer (around 40% of the time) compared to non–African American women of any age (around 15% of the time).

10. Is there anything I can do to prevent breast cancer? What about preventing triple negative breast cancer?

Primary prevention

Any treatment method or lifestyle change that directly prevents cancer cells from forming, growing, or multiplying.

Most of the associated risk factors cannot be controlled, therefore there are no means of **primary prevention**; that is, there's no vaccine or drug specifically targeted at breast cancer that can make it certain you won't get it. In high-risk women, drugs that target the estrogen receptor (i.e., tamoxifen) are sometimes used for preventing estrogen receptor positive breast cancer. However, no medicines have been proven to specifically prevent triple negative breast cancer.

Secondary prevention

Treatments or lifestyle changes that limit a person's exposure to cancer risk factors, but don't directly prevent the formation of cancer.

Secondary prevention (limiting the impact of factors you can control, as well as screening for cancer), early detection, and appropriate treatment early in the disease process can help to increase your chances of survival and complete cure should you get cancer. Secondary prevention includes breast self-exams beginning around age 20 years and consideration of screening mammography starting at age 40 years, depending on your other risk factors. If you have very high risk features, you may need to begin breast cancer screening even before age 40. Based on identified risk factors, promoting breastfeeding and maintaining a healthy weight through diet and exercise are also strategies to consider.

PART THREE

Inherited Breast Cancer

Is triple negative breast cancer inherited? How do genes affect the risk of being diagnosed with triple negative breast cancer?

What is the *BRCA* gene, and how is it related to triple negative breast cancer?

If I'm concerned about being a *BRCA* mutation carrier, how would I get tested?

More . . .

11. Is triple negative breast cancer inherited? How do genes affect the risk of being diagnosed with triple negative breast cancer?

Patients with breast cancer, even triple negative breast cancer, may have very different family histories. For instance, one woman with triple negative breast cancer may have had a mother, maternal aunt, and sister all with triple negative breast cancer, each diagnosed at a younger age and prior to menopause. The next woman may be the first in her family to be diagnosed with breast cancer of any type. Thus, every woman's experience with breast cancer is different and her risk for inheriting breast cancer is also individual. Although not always the case, families with several generations of breast cancer, especially breast cancers diagnosed at younger ages, appear at higher risk of inheriting their breast cancer.

It is estimated that only 8% (5–10%) of breast cancers of any type are the result of an identified and inherited **gene mutation**. Some genes do not function properly because there is a "mistake" in them. If a gene has a mistake, it is considered **mutated**, or altered. Such mutations are not at all unusual; in fact, all people have altered forms of some genes, and most of them are harmless. Some alterations, however, can increase your risk for certain illnesses, such as breast cancer. Mutations in genes may be inherited or may simply happen to a cell during a person's lifetime. In recent years, gene alterations have been found in some families with a history of breast cancer. Some women in these families also have had ovarian cancer. So, yes, triple negative breast cancer may be inherited in some women, but may be a completely sporadic (non-inherited) event in others. In either case, gene mutations either inherited

Gene mutation

An abnormality in genetic material that is either inherited or acquired; gene mutations can lead to cancer.

Mutated

Altered.

Triple negative breast cancer may be inherited in some women, but may be a completely sporadic (non-inherited) event in others.

or random appear to be related to the occurrence of triple negative breast cancer.

12. What is the BRCA gene, and how is it related to triple negative breast cancer?

As mentioned in the previous question, inherited alterations in specific genes are linked to about 8% (5–10%) of all breast cancers. These alterations are most commonly found in genes named *BRCA1* and *BRCA2* (BReast CAncer gene 1 and BReast CAncer gene 2). The normal version of these genes does not harm its carrier, but abnormal *BRCA1* and *BRCA2* genes are associated with higher rates of breast and/or ovarian cancer. It is estimated that the lifetime risk of developing breast cancer is 55% to 85% for BRCA1 and 50% to 85% for BRCA2 mutation carriers. Ovarian cancer lifetime risks range from 35% to 45% for BRCA1 and 15% to 25% for BRCA2 mutation carriers.

Both men and women have *BRCA1* and *BRCA2* genes, so alterations in these genes can be passed down from either the mother or the father. Although a woman with a *BRCA1* or *BRCA2* alteration is statistically more likely to develop breast and/or ovarian cancer than a woman without an alteration, not every woman who has an altered *BRCA1* or *BRCA2* gene will get breast or ovarian cancer. Genes are not the only factor that affects cancer risk, so an altered gene is not sufficient to cause cancer, and most cases of breast cancer do not involve an altered *BRCA1* or *BRCA2* gene.

Although not a "hard-and-fast" rule, patients with mutations in the *BRCA1* gene who do develop breast cancer usually develop triple negative breast cancer, while those with *BRCA2* mutations tend to develop estrogen receptor- and/or progesterone receptor-positive breast cancers. Studies have shown that among certain groups of women with triple negative breast cancer, as many as 20% of these women have mutations in the *BRCA1* gene. Although this is a much higher risk than 8% among all patients with breast cancer, not all triple negative breast cancers are associated with an abnormal *BRCA1* gene. It is important to talk to your doctor about your particular family history and individual risk for having a mutation in either the *BRCA1* or *BRCA2* mutation. If you and your doctor feel it is appropriate, the next step would be meeting with a genetic counselor to discuss your risk and need for gene mutation testing.

13. If I'm concerned about being a BRCA mutation carrier, how would I get tested?

Again, it is very important to talk to your doctor about your family history and potential risk for inheriting breast cancer through a gene mutation (i.e., *BRCA*). If you and your doctor discuss your risk and decide genetic testing is right for you, the next step is meeting with a board-certified genetic counselor. During this consultation, you and the genetic counselor will construct a **"family tree"** outlining all of your family members who have had a diagnosis of cancer, their kind of cancer, and their age at diagnosis. Thus, it is very important that you come to this consultation with as much knowledge about your family history as possible. This summary will help you and the genetic counselor determine your risk for a gene mutation and decide if genetic testing is right for you. If you decide to move forward with testing, you will provide a blood sample for gene testing. A specialized laboratory will look for

Family tree

A diagram of a family's ancestry.

alterations in genes known to increase the risk for breast cancer, specifically *BRCA1* and *BRCA2*. It should take several weeks to process the test results.

14. If I do have a mutation in either the BRCA1 or BRCA2 gene, how will I be notified?

Once the results of your tests are complete, you will be contacted by your doctor or the genetic counseling group with whom you initially met. You will be told if you have a mutation in a gene (i.e., *BRCA1* or *BRCA2*) that may have contributed to your risk of breast cancer. You will also receive counseling and detailed information on what this test means for you and your family members and how the results should be interpreted. This information will also be given to your doctor so you can discuss the results with him or her, as well.

15. If I'm diagnosed with a BRCA1 or BRCA2 mutation, how might the treatment options for my triple negative breast cancer differ?

If you are diagnosed with a mutation in either the *BRCA1* or *BRCA2* genes at the same time as a triple negative breast cancer, the treatment of your current breast cancer will likely remain very similar to treatment assuming you did not have a gene mutation. You will, however, be given options about **prophylactic surgeries**—surgeries to reduce the risk of another breast cancer or a new ovarian cancer developing. These surgeries might include **bilateral prophylactic mastectomies**, which is the removal of noncancerous normal breast tissue to reduce the risk of another breast cancer in the future, or **bilateral prophylactic salpingo-oophorectomy (BSO)**, which is the removal

Prophylactic surgeries

Surgeries to reduce the risk of another breast cancer or a new ovarian cancer from developing.

Bilateral prophylactic mastectomies

Removal of noncancerous normal breast tissue to reduce the risk of another breast cancer in the future.

Bilateral prophylactic salpingo-oophorectomy (BSO)

Removal of both ovaries and fallopian tubes to prevent a future ovarian cancer.

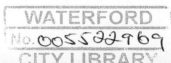

of both ovaries and fallopian tubes to prevent a future ovarian cancer. It is estimated that prophylactic mastectomies reduce the risk of breast cancer by 90% and prophylactic salpingo-oophorectomy reduces the risk of future ovarian cancer by greater than 90% among patients with **BRCA mutations**. Of course, these options are highly individualized, and patients are encouraged to talk these options over with their doctors, genetic counselors, and families before proceeding. Prophylactic surgeries are generally delayed until after the age of 35 years and childbearing is complete.

Another option to discuss with your doctor is increased surveillance. This would involve the following:

- Intensive breast screening in the form of annual **bilateral breast magnetic resonance imaging (MRI)** and bilateral mammograms starting at age 25 years (or individualized based on family history)
- Monthly breast self-exam starting at age 18 years
- Clinical breast exam two to four times annually starting at age 25 years
- Twice-yearly ovarian cancer screening with ultrasound and serum CA-125 levels beginning at age 35 years among *BRCA* mutation carriers with intact breasts and ovaries

Some women with *BRCA* mutations opt for **chemoprevention,** which involves taking medicines, namely the selective estrogen receptor modulator (SERM) **tamoxifen,** to reduce the risk of breast cancer. While tamoxifen has been shown to reduce the risk of contralateral breast cancer (the opposite side of prior breast cancer) by as much as 50% regardless of estrogen receptor status, the role of tamoxifen in *BRCA* mutation carriers with triple negative breast cancers is much less clear.

BRCA mutations

Mutations in either the *BRCA1 or 2* gene that leads to inherited breast cancer.

Bilateral breast magnetic resonance imaging (MRI)

A non-invasive medical imaging technique used to visualize soft tissue structures, including the bilateral breasts.

Chemoprevention

Medicines prescribed to prevent cancers.

Tamoxifen

A drug used to treat breast cancers that express the estrogen and/or progesterone receptors, called a selective estrogen receptor modulator (SERM).

16. I'm worried that I'll lose my insurance if I'm found to have a mutation in the BRCA1 or BRCA2 gene. Is this possible?

The Genetic Information Nondiscrimination Act of 2008 (GINA) is a new federal law that protects Americans from being treated unfairly because of differences in their DNA that may affect their health. Hence, genetic testing will not affect health insurance coverage. The new law prevents discrimination from health insurers and employers. The part of the law relating to health insurers took effect May 2009, and those relating to employers, November 2009. The law was needed to help ease concerns about discrimination that might keep some people from getting genetic tests that could benefit their health. The law also enables people to take part in research studies without fear that their DNA information might be used against them in health insurance or the workplace. The law protects people from discrimination by health insurers and employers on the basis of DNA information. The law does not cover members of the military. In addition, the law does not cover life insurance, disability insurance, and long-term care insurance. Before the federal law was passed, many states had passed laws against genetic discrimination. The degree of protection from these laws varies widely among the different states. The federal law sets a minimum standard of protection that must be met in all states. It does not weaken the protections provided by any state law.

If you are thinking about genetic testing, be sure to talk with your doctor, a genetic counselor, or other health professionals, and take some time to get answers to your questions (see the following sample questions). You may want to get more than one opinion. For more information on genetic testing or for a referral to centers that have healthcare professionals trained in genetics, call the National Cancer Institute's Cancer Information Service at 1-800-4-CANCER. The Cancer Information Service can also provide information about clinical trials and research studies.

Examples of questions you might have include:

- What are the chances that a gene alteration is involved in the cancer in my family?
- What are my chances of having an altered gene?
- Besides altered *BRCA1* or *BRCA2* genes, what are other risk factors for breast and ovarian cancers?
- Are all genetic tests the same? How much does the test cost? How long will it take to get my results?
- What are the possible results of the test?
- What would a positive result mean for me?
- What would a negative result mean for me?
- How might a positive test result affect my health insurance? Life insurance? Employment?
- Do I want to submit my test results to an insurance company? If so will they pay for the testing?

PART FOUR

Diagnosis

How is triple negative breast cancer diagnosed, and what symptoms should I bring to my doctor's attention?

If I have breast symptoms, what tests might be done?

If I am diagnosed with breast cancer, how will we know it is triple negative?

More . . .

17. How is triple negative breast cancer diagnosed, and what symptoms should I bring to my doctor's attention?

Women with triple negative breast cancer can come to medical attention in a few different ways. The most common way is when a woman feels a new lump in her breast. Other women first come to medical attention because of an abnormality on a routine mammogram.

If you note a new or changing lump in your breast, the best advice is to consult your doctor or nurse.

If you note a new or changing lump in your breast, the best advice is to consult your doctor or nurse. Most of the time, breast lumps turn out to be benign (non-cancerous). However, it is important not to ignore a new lump. Your healthcare provider will carefully examine your breast, including the lump and the surrounding breast tissue. He or she will also examine your skin and the lymph nodes under your arm. Depending on what is found, your doctor may recommend further testing and/or follow-up.

Other symptoms you should bring to your doctor's attention are redness of the skin of the breast, swelling and pain in the breast (especially if it is more concentrated on one side than the other), bleeding from the nipple, nipple inversion (your nipple starts pointing inward instead of outward), swelling or lumps in the underarm areas, or any other significant change from your usual pattern.

18. If I have breast symptoms, what tests might be done?

Imaging

The most common imaging test is a mammogram, which uses X-rays to look at the structures of the breast. Cancers may appear as either calcium deposits (white flecks or branching lines), as a solid-appearing lump, or as "architectural distortion," meaning that there looks to be tethering or pulling of the surrounding normal breast tissue. Your doctor might also order an ultrasound, which uses sound waves to determine whether a lump is solid or filled with fluid.

Biopsy

Your doctor will assess your need for a biopsy based upon your age, your symptoms, his or her examination of your breast, and results of the imaging tests just described. The purpose of a biopsy is to try to obtain some cells to look at under the microscope in order to determine whether cancer is present.

There are several different ways to do a biopsy.

Core Needle Biopsy

This is the most common type of breast biopsy. Before the biopsy, numbing medicine similar to Novocain is usually injected to reduce the pain and discomfort associated with the procedure. A needle is used to remove a few small cylinders of tissue for analysis.

A core needle biopsy can be done in the office with the doctor directly palpating (feeling) the lump, or it can be done with ultrasound guidance, meaning that the doctor can locate the mass with the ultrasound machine and aim the needle directly at the lump. Sometimes, the lump or imaging abnormality cannot be felt accurately and cannot be seen on ultrasound. Under those circumstances, a core needle biopsy can sometimes still be done, either with stereotactic guidance (a special mammography machine that allows the radiologist to direct the needle to the area of abnormality) or with breast MRI guidance (see Question 23 for more on breast MRI).

Diagnosis

After the procedure, you will be allowed to go home. Some patients experience pain and bruising around the biopsy site for a few days to a week or so afterward. In addition, many patients find that the lump feels "bigger" after the biopsy. This is almost never because of cancer growth; rather, it is related to some bleeding and scar tissue formation at the site of the biopsy.

Often, you will not receive a diagnosis on the same day, but your doctor will call a few days later to review the results.

Fine Needle Aspiration

Fine needle aspiration (FNA) uses a very thin needle to sample fluid or cells from a mass for evaluation. FNA can be used in several situations. For example, when the radiologist suspects that the mass could be a benign cyst, FNA can be used to remove the fluid inside the cyst. Depending on whether the cyst disappears completely or not, and your doctor's level of concern about your symptoms, you may be advised to have a repeat physical examination and imaging studies in a few months for follow-up. Or, you may be advised to proceed to a core needle biopsy. FNA can also be used in some situations to obtain a sample of enlarged lymph nodes to determine prior to surgery whether the lymph nodes contain cancer. However, because the amount of tissue obtained using FNA is smaller than with a core needle biopsy, core needle biopsy is the preferred type of biopsy in most situations when breast cancer is suspected.

As with core needle biopsy, FNA can be done in the office with the doctor directly palpating the lump, or it can be done with ultrasound guidance, meaning that the doctor can locate the mass with the ultrasound machine and aim the needle directly at the lump.

After the procedure, you will be allowed to go home. Often, you will not receive a diagnosis on the same day, but your doctor will call a few days later to review the results.

Incisional/Excisional Biopsy

Sometimes it is not possible to safely or accurately obtain a core needle biopsy or fine needle aspiration. For example, if you have a lump at the very back of your breast, close to your ribs, your doctor might be concerned about the safety of obtaining a needle biopsy because of the risk of lung damage or other possible risks. Or, the lump might not show up on the imaging tests at all, and your doctor may be concerned that he or she might not be able to obtain a good biopsy sample using the previously described techniques. Or, the results of a core needle biopsy may not be definitive.

In these cases, your doctor might recommend either an incisional (a portion of the lump is removed) or excisional (the entire mass is removed) biopsy in the operating room. Incisional and excisional biopsies are more like regular surgery. You will typically receive local anesthesia (similar to Novocain) in the area of the biopsy as well as IV medications to make you drowsy. An incision is made to remove a piece of tissue for analysis. Stitches will be placed to close the incision, and you will spend some time being monitored in the recovery room afterward.

After the procedure, you will be allowed to go home. Often, you will not receive a diagnosis on the same day, but your doctor will call a few days later to review the results.

19. If I am diagnosed with breast cancer, how will we know it is triple negative?

After you have a biopsy, your tissue specimen will be carefully examined by a pathologist. A pathologist is a doctor who has special training in distinguishing between normal, precancerous, and cancerous cells on the basis of their appearance under the microscope.

One of the first tasks of the pathologist is to determine whether the biopsy shows cancer. This depends on the appearance of the cells as well as the pattern of the cells (the architecture). Triple negative cancers almost always fall under the classification of "invasive ductal carcinoma," meaning the cells and architecture appear cancerous ("invasive") and have an appearance similar to breast ducts. Triple negative cancers are also usually high grade or poorly differentiated, meaning they look aggressive under the microscope.

After making a diagnosis of breast cancer, the pathologist will order additional tests to determine the breast cancer subtype. Specifically, the pathologist will examine the results of three tests: estrogen receptor (ER), progesterone receptor (PR), and HER2. The term *triple negative* breast cancer comes from the fact that the breast cancer is negative for all three tests. That is, it is estrogen receptor-negative, progesterone receptor-negative, and HER2-negative. Because of the extra testing involved, it may take up to 1 to 2 weeks after your biopsy for you and your doctor to know whether your cancer is triple negative.

Special Tumor Types

It is important to note that there are some very rare breast cancer subtypes that are estrogen receptor-negative, progesterone receptor-negative, and HER2-negative, but that do not behave like typical triple negative breast cancers. For example, adenoid cystic carcinomas of the breast, which account for only about 1 in 1000 breast cancers, are negative for all three markers, but have an excellent prognosis, even without **chemotherapy**. These cancers appear different under the microscope, compared to typical, triple negative breast cancer. Because this diagnosis is so uncommon, and because the recommended treatment can be quite different, if you are diagnosed with adenoid cystic carcinoma or another rare breast cancer tumor type, it may be helpful to seek a second opinion to confirm the diagnosis and treatment plan.

Chemotherapy

The use of chemical agents (drugs) to systemically treat cancer.

20. Will my doctor tell me if I have triple negative breast cancer, or should I ask?

More and more often, your doctor will tell you what type of breast cancer you have. Your doctor will most likely discuss whether your cancer is estrogen receptor-positive or -negative, because this influences whether hormonal treatments (e.g., tamoxifen) will be effective. Your doctor will also most likely discuss whether your cancer is HER2-positive or -negative, because this influences whether medicines like Herceptin (trastuzumab) might be helpful. If your cancer is triple negative, then neither hormonal treatments nor Herceptin are helpful, and they are not recommended. In general, if your cancer is triple negative, your doctor will be somewhat more likely to recommend some amount of traditional chemotherapy, even if you have stage I disease, unless the tumor is very small or you have other serious medical problems.

Diagnosis

21. I had my mammogram every year as instructed by my primary care physician, but I was diagnosed with a triple negative breast cancer anyway. How is this possible?

In comparison to the more common type of breast cancer (i.e., estrogen receptor-positive breast cancer), triple negative breast cancers more often appear as "interval cancers," meaning they can show up between regular mammograms. In fact, some studies have shown that the majority of triple negative breast cancers are first detected when a woman feels a lump in her breast. The reasons for this are not completely clear; however, there are several possible theories. First, triple negative breast cancers tend to grow somewhat faster, so that they might not have been present or may have been too small to show up on your previous mammogram. Second, some studies have suggested that triple negative breast cancers might be less commonly associated with calcifications (calcium deposits), which can show up easily on a mammogram and are often the first sign that a cancer or precancer might be present.

Even if your previous mammogram was negative, when you present to your doctor with a new lump, it is very likely that he or she will want to obtain another mammogram. Sometimes once a lump appears, it is then visible on the mammogram and there can be other useful information gained at that time.

In some cases, a woman finds a new lump in her breast but the mammogram still does not show anything abnormal. The doctor may then order an ultrasound and/or a breast MRI test to further evaluate the lump. It is important to note that even if your cancer does not show up on a mammogram, your doctor will still recommend that you be followed with yearly mammograms after you complete your breast cancer treatment. This is because mammograms have a long track record of increasing the chance of early detection of breast cancer and may still detect new problems going forward.

22. What other tests, other than my breast biopsy, may be needed following a diagnosis of triple negative breast cancer?

After a diagnosis of triple negative breast cancer, your doctor may order additional tests to help guide the next steps in your care. Guidelines for additional testing have been put forth by the National Comprehensive Cancer Network (NCCN) and other professional organizations.

Your doctor will first take a careful medical history, including breast cancer risk factors and family history. Your doctor will also ask you a series of questions about your overall health and any other symptoms you might have, such as bone pain, liver or abdominal pain, cough, or shortness of breath. Finally, your doctor will perform a physical examination. The physical examination will include listening to your heart and lungs, feeling your liver, palpating (feeling) the breast mass, examining the skin overlying the breast, and feeling for any enlarged or suspicious lymph nodes. If you have not already had mammograms of both breasts, this will be performed. Your doctor will also talk to you about whether a breast MRI is necessary (see Question 23).

If your doctor suspects you have either stage I or stage II breast cancer, then you may have blood tests such as a complete blood count, liver function tests, and an alkaline phosphatase test (this is a test that looks at

Mammograms have a long track record of increasing the chance of early detection of breast cancer.

Diagnosis

both liver function and bone problems). If the results of these tests are normal and if you don't have any other concerning symptoms, you will most likely not need additional scans or tests to work up your breast cancer.

If your doctor suspects you have stage III breast cancer (for example, if he or she feels multiple enlarged lymph nodes or if you have inflammatory breast cancer), then you may have blood tests such as a complete blood count, liver function tests, and an alkaline phosphatase test. Your doctor will also order tests such as a bone scan to make sure the cancer has not spread to your bones as well as tests to look at your lungs and liver. The types of tests vary from doctor to doctor; common tests include a combination of a chest X-ray to look at the lungs with an ultrasound test to look at the liver, or, alternatively, a computed tomography (CT) scan to look at your lungs and liver at the same time.

You will then meet separately with an anesthesiologist to discuss your upcoming breast surgery. Sometimes additional preoperative tests must be done to maximize the safety of surgery (for example, a chest X-ray or heart tests if you are older and have a history of significant heart problems). Your doctor will discuss with you which tests will be required.

Finally, regardless of what stage of breast cancer your doctor suspects you might have, if you have concerning symptoms, then your doctor will order tests targeted at those symptoms. For example, if you have suspicious bone pains or abnormal blood tests suspicious for cancer in the bones, your doctor will order a bone scan. If you have abnormal liver function tests, an enlarged liver on physical examination, or other concerning abdominal symptoms, your doctor might order scans of your abdomen. If you have shortness of breath or a nagging cough, your doctor might order either a chest X-ray or a CT scan of your chest.

Typically, results of these tests may take up to a week to be available. When your doctor orders these tests, you will also be given a plan of how the results will be communicated to you (e.g., in person, over the telephone).

You should know that it is quite uncommon for women to have stage IV (metastatic) breast cancer when they first present with a breast lump. In fact, on average, the chance of finding stage IV breast cancer is less than 10%. This number is even lower still in women with small tumors and women without enlarged lymph nodes. Therefore, if your doctor does recommend additional tests, fortunately, chances are that the tests will not show any evidence of cancer spread to distant organs (e.g., liver, lung, bone).

23. I have had a mammogram; will I need a breast MRI?

Magnetic resonance imaging (MRI) is a technique that uses a strong magnet to produce images of your breast(s). Because it takes pictures in a different way than either mammogram or ultrasound, it can be useful in some situations to help your doctor guide your care. However, it is important to note that MRI is not a replacement for mammograms. Rather, it can be a useful supplement, in addition to mammography, for detecting and staging breast cancer.

One important downside of breast MRI is that in addition to detecting breast cancer, it can also show

One important downside of breast MRI is that in addition to detecting breast cancer, it can also show many benign (noncancerous) findings.

many benign (noncancerous) findings. It can some-times be hard to tell the difference between cancerous and noncancerous findings on the MRI. This can lead to additional testing and anxiety. Breast MRI has not been proven to improve your chances of survival. So, unlike mammograms, which are a very important part of your breast cancer work-up and should be per-formed in nearly all circumstances, not all women need to have a breast MRI as part of their breast cancer workup. Your doctor will discuss with you whether an MRI is recommended for you.

There are several situations in which MRI might be considered.

As part of the initial work-up of a new breast cancer diag-nosis: If you have undergone a breast biopsy and have just been diagnosed with breast cancer, your doctor might order a breast MRI under certain circumstances, such as the following:

- Your doctor suspects there may be multiple tumors in your breast.
- Your doctor is concerned that the mammogram or ultrasound is not showing the full extent of your cancer.
- Your doctor would like additional assessment of the size and/or extent of your cancer to help in planning surgery.

As part of assessment in patients receiving pre-operative chemotherapy: In some situations, your doctor may rec-ommend that you receive chemotherapy prior to hav-ing surgery. For example, if you have a large tumor, giving chemotherapy before surgery may shrink the tumor and allow you to have a lumpectomy instead of a mastectomy. If your doctor recommends pre-operative chemotherapy, he or she may also recommend you have a breast MRI before and after finishing chemotherapy to check how well the treatment worked and to help plan the most appropriate surgery.

As part of routine follow-up: If you have been diagnosed with breast cancer, then, after you have completed your treatments, you will be followed closely for recurrences of your breast cancer and for new breast cancers. The American Cancer Society has issued guidelines to help women and their doctors understand when breast MRI may be useful as part of follow-up care.

Breast MRI is recommended once a year if:

- You carry a mutation in either the *BRCA1* or *BRCA2* gene
- You are a first-degree relative of a *BRCA1* or *BRCA2* carrier, but have chosen not to be tested yourself
- You have a very high (20–25%) lifetime risk of developing breast cancer
- You received significant radiation treatments to your chest between ages 10 and 30 years (for example, if you were treated with chest radiation for lymphoma)
- You have another inherited genetic reason for breast cancer (These are rare and include Li-Fraumeni syndrome and Cowden syndrome.)

Breast MRI is not recommended if you are at average risk (i.e., <15% lifetime risk) of breast cancer.

If you don't fall into any of the categories listed here, then your doctor will discuss with you, with respect to your specific situation, whether MRI is right for you as part of your follow-up care. Some of the factors you and your doctor may consider are your age, family history, and breast density.

24. My doctor has recommended a breast MRI. What should I expect?

If your doctor recommends a breast MRI, you will be asked a series of questions to maximize the chance that the test will be safe. For example, you will be asked if you have a pacemaker, cochlear (ear) implant, artificial heart valve, shrapnel, or other metal objects or electronic devices in your body. You will be asked if you could possibly be pregnant. Although MRI can be done if you are pregnant, you and your doctor will want to carefully weigh the potential risks and benefits of the test ahead of time.

If you have claustrophobia (i.e., you are afraid of enclosed spaces), your doctor may give you a prescription for an antianxiety pill to take prior to the test. Let your doctor know in advance if this is a concern for you.

On the day of the test, you will be asked to remove all metal and electronic objects (such as jewelry, watches, etc.) before the test. Usually, a breast MRI is done with an intravenous (IV) dye. A technician or nurse will place an IV in your arm. You will then be asked to lie face-down on your stomach and will enter the MRI machine. The MRI machine looks like a large tunnel with a moveable table that can slide in and out of the center. You will be asked to lie very still on the table during the test, which usually takes between 40 and 60 minutes. During the test, you will hear clanging and thumping sounds. Some centers offer earplugs to patients or play music to help patients relax during the test. After the test is over, the IV will be removed and you will be allowed to go home.

Usually MRI results will not be available right away. It usually takes several days to one week for your doctor to receive the results.

Diagnosis

PART FIVE

Treatment for Early-Stage Triple Negative Breast Cancer

I've just been diagnosed with triple negative breast cancer. What do I do now?

What is radiation therapy?

What sort of things will my doctor be considering when selecting systemic treatments like chemotherapy to treat my triple negative breast cancer?

More . . .

GENERAL TREATMENT QUESTIONS

25. I've just been diagnosed with triple negative breast cancer. What do I do now?

A diagnosis of cancer of any kind can be quite scary and difficult to accept. It is important to recognize that the first few days to weeks after receiving a cancer diagnosis of any kind can be especially anxiety-producing and unsettling. Not only are you facing your own fears about being diagnosed with cancer, but you are also likely juggling how this diagnosis affects your family life, your work life, and your day-to-day routine. You are also getting a "crash course" in the basics of breast cancer, meeting lots of new people, and possibly having invasive procedures (e.g., breast biopsies), all while juggling your already busy life. This period of uncertainty will subside as you and your doctors put together your treatment plan. Although you are likely in a state of shock after receiving your breast cancer diagnosis, it is important that you not wait too long to start treatments. Here are a few suggestions of ways to make the first few days to weeks more tolerable after receiving a diagnosis of triple negative breast cancer.

Call on your family and friends. It is likely that you will have difficulty remembering all the information you receive from your doctors and medical team. Patients find it very helpful to bring their spouses, close family members, or friends to their initial evaluations with their breast cancer care team. Having two pairs of ears is always better than one. It is also helpful for you to have this partner take notes about the conversation or even tape record the conversation so you can listen to it again when you are not feeling so anxious or overwhelmed.

Educate yourself—a little at a time. The fact that you are reading this book is a step in the right direction. Often the unknown is more disturbing than the known. Although you are certainly not expected to become an oncologist, knowing what to expect about your breast cancer diagnosis and upcoming treatments can "demystify" the situation so you will know what to expect. Pace yourself as you educate yourself and try not to become overwhelmed by the vast amount of information available. It is also important to talk to your doctors and research team to know if the information you are gathering is sound. There are many resources listed in the appendix (e.g., from the National Cancer Institute, American Cancer Society, Susan G. Komen Foundation, Triple Negative Breast Cancer Foundation, Young Survival Coalition) that you may find beneficial. Also, be sure to visit the patient resource center at your doctor's office, if available, to find resources (and/or support groups) in your community.

Talk to others in a similar situation. Many patients find it comforting to share their experiences with women facing similar emotions and going through similar treatments. It is not uncommon to feel like family and friends without cancer "just can't understand." Talking to others in your shoes can be quite beneficial. This sort of dialogue can come in the form of support groups in your community, one-on-one interactions with patients in your community, and/or online breast cancer-oriented chat groups. Think about what may be most beneficial to fit your personality. If you are feeling quite overwhelmed (i.e., having difficulty with anxiety, depression, or insomnia), talk to your doctor about psychological resources in your community and within your own cancer center.

Patient comment:

I found that some family and friends turned away from me. One said it was my fault, others just avoided talking or being around me. On top of the diagnosis, emotions are raw, people react differently to you, and you can have a feeling of isolation. I found an online support group that helped me from feeling so isolated and I was able to discuss with others who understood what having breast cancer was all about. Then I found the TNBCF website/forum where finally I could be with women who had TNBC, even better because of its focus on just TNBC.

I personally found educating myself through reliable online resources to be significant for me. I feel knowledge works in our favor. After going through a cancer journey more than once, you learn pretty quickly that advocating for yourself is important. I felt empowered to ask questions, participate in my care, and to know to some degree what was happening.

26. Now that I have a diagnosis of triple negative breast cancer, I'm ready to get started with treatment. What are my options?

There are many treatment options available for breast cancer. Although some aspects of the treatment of triple negative breast cancer may differ from breast cancer in general, many remain the same. We will review the basics of some of the common treatments here.

Mastectomy

Surgical removal of the whole breast.

Lumpectomy

Only the tumor and a small section of normal breast tissue are removed from the breast, leaving the breast virtually intact.

Surgery. **Mastectomy** and/or **lumpectomy** involves the surgical removal of the cancerous tissue and a certain amount of the surrounding tissue as well as nodes from the nearby lymphatic system. The extent of surgery is determined by the type and extent of the cancer, and it may or may not be accompanied by other types of therapy. Surgery can also include a sentinel node biopsy, involving removal of the lymph nodes nearest the breast, or an axillary lymph node dissection, in which multiple lymph nodes are removed if there is evidence that the cancer has already spread there.

Radiation. Radiation therapy incorporates the use of high-energy X-rays to kill cancer cells and shrink tumors. Radiation may come from a machine outside the body (external radiation therapy) or from inserting materials that produce radiation (radioisotopes) into the area where the cancer cells are found through thin plastic tubes (internal radiation therapy).

Chemotherapy. Chemotherapy uses drugs to systemically treat cancer. These drugs are provided either orally or intravenously. Chemotherapy will be discussed in further detail in later sections of this book.

Targeted therapy. Targeted therapies are designed to take advantage of differences between cancerous cells and normal cells in your body. Some examples of targeted therapies used in breast cancer are hormonal therapy and trastuzumab (Herceptin).

Hormonal therapy (which includes drugs like tamoxifen and/or an aromatase inhibitor) is not used in the treatment of triple negative breast cancer. Triple negative breast cancer does not express the estrogen and/or progesterone receptor on its cell surface; therefore this type of breast cancer is not responsive to manipulation of these receptors. Perhaps the most well-known example of targeted therapy to treat breast cancer is that of **trastuzumab** (Herceptin), a monoclonal antibody that binds to the HER2 receptor on breast cancer cells. As discussed earlier, triple negative breast cancer does not express HER2 on its cell surface; thus this type of breast cancer is not effectively treated with

Treatment for Early-Stage Triple Negative Breast Cancer

Targeted therapy
Treatment that targets specific molecules involved in carcinogenesis or tumor growth.

Hormonal therapy
Treatment that blocks the effects of hormones upon cancers that depend on hormones to grow (also referred to as endocrine therapy).

Trastuzumab (Herceptin)
An anti-cancer drug that targets breast cancers that express the HER2 protein.

Anti-angiogenic agents

An anti-cancer drugs that block blood vessel formation around and inside tumors.

PARP inhibitors

An anti-cancer agents that block a tumor's ability to repair DNA damage.

No one doctor is able to provide all of the care and service you may need, so it's necessary to use a team of specialists to look at your case from different perspectives.

trastuzumab. Other types of targeted therapies that affect the growth of blood vessels that feed tumors (**anti-angiogenic agents**) and those that block DNA repair (**PARP inhibitors**) appear promising in the treatment of advanced triple negative breast cancer and will be discussed in later sections of this book.

27. When I was diagnosed with triple negative breast cancer, I thought I would be seen by one breast cancer doctor. Who are all of these specialists and what are their roles?

Breast cancer is a complex disease. No one doctor is able to provide all of the care and service you may need, so it's necessary to use a team of specialists to look at your case from different perspectives. When you are first diagnosed with breast cancer, your primary care doctor or gynecologist will typically take the role of directing your initial testing and referring you to the appropriate specialists. With the advice of these experts, he or she will help guide you through the many steps in your care. Often, once a diagnosis has been made, your medical oncologist will become your "point person" in coordinating your breast cancer treatment and follow-up. You should still continue to follow-up with your primary care doctor for your other health needs.

The following medical experts may be part of your team:

> *Primary care doctor.* This is your general care physician, the person who gives you regular checkups and is likely the person who helped to diagnose you through either physical exam or breast imaging. If your primary care doctor is trained in gynecology, he or she may also act as the manager and main source of information among your treatment team

members and you. If not, you may ask him or her to consult with the team if you feel more comfortable having a familiar person on board. Often the presence of someone you know well on your team can be reassuring.

Gynecologist. This doctor is a specialist in women's health. If your primary care doctor is not a gynecologist, this specialist may manage the team's information, possibly jointly with your primary physician. If you have your own gynecologist who performs your regular exams, you may prefer to ask him or her to perform this function.

Radiologist. Generally the same doctor who reads your mammogram, the radiologist is part of the team because additional X-rays, such as bone scans or chest films, could be needed to determine the exact stage of your cancer. The radiologist may have also performed your first breast biopsy that confirmed your diagnosis of triple negative breast cancer. The radiologist will not necessarily be directly involved in your treatment, but his or her input is required in determining what the correct treatment should be.

Surgical oncologist. This cancer specialist performs biopsies and other surgical procedures, such as removing a lump (lumpectomy) or a breast (mastectomy).

Oncologist or medical oncologist. This cancer specialist will gather all of the information about your case to help determine your treatment choices, including how long, how much, and what types of systemic therapies are best for you.

Radiation oncologist. This cancer specialist determines the amount of radiotherapy required. Not all patients require radiation, so not all teams will include a radiation oncologist.

Plastic surgeon. This surgical specialist will perform any reconstruction procedures that might be required either during or after your breast surgery. This specialist will consult with the oncologists on your team to determine the best timing of such procedures.

Nutritionist. This health professional with specialized training in nutrition can offer help with choices about the foods you eat. Because of the effects that some treatments can have on appetite and nutritional status, it can be important to assess and supplement your diet during cancer treatment.

In most cases, your primary care physician and/or gynecologist will recommend qualified doctors for each of the positions on your team. Many people simply accept the doctors their primary physician recommends, and if you are comfortable with those choices, then you need not look further than your doctor's recommendations. Because the surgeon usually will be responsible for the first portion of your treatment, it is important that you meet him or her and feel comfortable with his or her qualifications and abilities. The American Board of Medical Specialties (ABMS) certifies specialists, and verification of the physician's credentials can be obtained by visiting the ABMS Web site or calling their toll-free number (see the appendix).

If your primary care physician has no suggestions, or if you aren't comfortable with some of the doctors recommended, your insurance company usually can provide a list of specialists in their database, and you may wish to choose one of these. Another option is to check the list of specialists available from your local chapter of the American Cancer Society or from the National Cancer Institute. There are also a number of online services that can help you to locate both physicians and hospitals accredited to treat your disease. Some even provide ratings as to which physicians and hospitals provide the best care. A list of these services is available in the appendix.

28. I have met with a group of doctors to discuss my treatment options. Should I also seek a second opinion?

After you meet with your team of doctors, you may feel completely satisfied with the information you received and ready to move on with treatment. You may, however, have unanswered questions or may simply want to hear another viewpoint on your treatment options for triple negative breast cancer. It is very common and normal to seek a second opinion, and telling your doctor you would like a second opinion should not offend him or her. Another opinion may help you confirm or adjust your treatment based on the diagnosis and stage of the disease and may also help ease your mind about your choice of treatment and decisions. Sometimes second-opinion doctors may provide information about a research study specifically tailored for women with triple negative breast cancer that may offer a new treatment method or clinical trial.

There are a number of ways you can obtain a second opinion. You can ask your doctor to refer you to another breast cancer specialist. If you are not comfortable with that, call the National Cancer Institute's Cancer Information Service (1-800-4-CANCER) for help in locating cancer specialists who may be in your area; also, talk with women in breast cancer organizations. Ask other women who have been through breast cancer treatment for referrals, keeping in mind that your recommended treatment may be different from theirs because not all breast cancer cases are the same.

29. What sort of things should I be thinking about when I select my treatment plan with my doctors?

When developing an individualized treatment plan for your triple negative breast cancer, many factors will need to be considered. These factors will include your age, menopausal status, general health (and ability to tolerate therapy safely), the location of the tumor, involvement of lymph nodes in the axilla (under the arm), tumor size, and breast size. In the case of triple negative breast cancer, therapies that target the estrogen and/or progesterone receptors or the HER2 protein will not be considered, as triple negative breast cancers lack expression of these key breast cancer features. Your doctor will discuss each of these issues with you and provide rationale for selected treatments.

From your perspective, you may also want to consider logistical details including distance of treatment facilities from your home, who can provide transportation given that many treatments you may receive may make you drowsy (and therefore unsafe to drive yourself home), and, if the treatment facility is not in your hometown, who you can rely on in a pinch (i.e., your primary care physician or local oncologist, who may have referred you to a larger facility for a specialized treatment). For younger women, future childbearing may also be a consideration, making discussions with **reproductive endocrinologists** and **infertility specialists** important *before* embarking on a chemotherapy treatment program (discussed in further detail in Part 6). Most doctors recommend that women who choose to

Reproductive endocrinologists

Doctors who help assess a patient's reproductive system and help the patient achieve a pregnancy.

Infertility specialist

A physician who helps women and/or couples achieve pregnancy.

have a family after a diagnosis of breast cancer wait at least 2 years following diagnosis so they can complete all of their recommended therapies. Two to three years following diagnosis is also the highest risk period for recurrence, for women with triple negative breast cancer. Your doctors want to ensure you will be healthy, in regard to your breast cancer, before trying to get pregnant.

30. My doctors continue to mention "stage" and "grade." What do these terms mean?

Cancers can be classified by **stage**, a measure of the size and extent of the cancer, and by **histologic grade**, which describes how quickly or slowly cancer cells are growing and multiplying under the microscope and how abnormal they appear. Both stage and grade will be considered in the development of your breast cancer treatment plan. Because the grading of cancers is a touch less complicated, we'll discuss grading first.

The histologic grade assigned to a tumor is a way for the pathologist examining the tumor to describe how cancerous cells are arranged in relation to one another and to describe some of the features of individual cells. Grading of cancers uses classification levels of 1 to 3. Grade 1 tumors consist of relatively slow-growing cancer cells that look a great deal like normal cells; these are called "well-differentiated" cells. Grade 2 ("moderately differentiated") and grade 3 ("poorly differentiated") designations describe cancer cells that are scattered in arrangement, abnormal in appearance, and more aggressive in their spread than grade 1 cancers. Grade 3 is the fastest growing and most abnormal type. Triple negative breast cancers are commonly grade 3.

Pathologists determine stage based upon the status of three areas of concern: (1) the size of the tumor,

Stage

A numerical determination of how far the cancer has progressed.

Histologic grade

Describes how slow or fast the cancer is growing and progressing from stage to stage.

(2) whether cancer is present in the lymph nodes, and (3) whether metastasis has occurred. The various categories of these areas, taken from the tumor-node-metastasis (TNM) classification system, are taken in combination to assign a stage. Stage is given as one of the following categories:

- *Stage 0* (early stage) indicates findings of ductal carcinoma in situ (DCIS), lobular carcinoma in situ (LCIS), or tumorless Paget disease. No invasive cancer is reported, and there are no signs of spread to lymph nodes or tissue beyond the breast.
- *Stage I* (early stage) means that cancer cells are not found in the lymph nodes, and the tumor is no more than 2 cm (less than an inch) across.
- *Stage II* (early stage) means that cancer has spread to 1–3 lymph nodes under the arm (axilla), and/or the tumor in the breast is 2 to 5 cm (1 to 2 inches) across. This stage is subdivided into stages IIA and IIB.
- *Stage III* (advanced stage) is also called locally advanced cancer. The tumor in the breast is usually large (more than 5 cm [2 inches] across), the cancer is extensive in axillary lymph nodes, or it has spread to other lymph node areas or to other tissues near the breast. Stage III cancers are also divided into three substages. Cancers designated as stage IIIA include large tumors, or any tumors with 4–9 positive lymph nodes, while stage IIIB is reserved for those cancers that have spread to the chest wall or skin, particularly those that have visible external symptoms such as an ulcer on the breast skin, edema, or "orange peel" appearance of the skin. Inflammatory breast cancer is a stage IIIB type of locally advanced breast cancer. Stage IIIC cancers involve 10 or more positive axillary lymph nodes or involvement of other lymph node areas in the region.

- *Stage IV* is metastatic cancer. Stage IV cancers have spread from the breast to other organs of the body, for example, the lung, liver, or bone.

Triple negative breast cancer can occur at any stage. Women with early-stage triple negative breast cancer (stage I–II) may have the option of breast-sparing surgery (lumpectomy) followed by radiation therapy as their primary local treatment, or they may have a mastectomy. These approaches are equally effective in treating early-stage breast cancer. The choice of breast-sparing surgery or mastectomy depends mostly on the size and location of the tumor, the size of the woman's breast, certain features of the mammogram, and how the woman feels about preserving her breast. With either approach, lymph nodes under the arm generally are sampled, except in stage 0 cases.

Chemotherapy is the mainstay of systemic therapy for triple negative breast cancer. Most women with stage I and stage II breast cancer will be offered chemotherapy before (neoadjuvant) or after surgery (adjuvant). Chemotherapy is given to treat the whole body to prevent the survival of small microscopic breast cancer cells, which may persist despite surgery, and to prevent metastases and recurrence.

Patients with stage III triple negative breast cancer will be offered both local treatment to remove or destroy the cancer in the breast and systemic treatment to stop the disease from spreading. The local treatment may be surgery and/or radiation therapy to the breast and axilla. The systemic treatment is usually limited to chemotherapy; it may be given before or after local therapy. In some cases, chemotherapy and radiation are given at the same time.

Women who have stage IV triple negative breast cancer are recommended to receive chemotherapy to shrink the tumor or destroy cancer cells throughout the body. They may have surgery or radiation therapy to control the cancer in the breast, but this is often not necessary. Radiation may also be useful to control tumors in other parts of the body (e.g., painful bony lesions). It is important to emphasize that although stage IV cancer is a very serious and incurable illness and has a worse prognosis than cancers caught prior to reaching this stage, women can enjoy a good quality of life after a diagnosis of metastatic cancer, and there are a number of new therapies available that have proven effective against metastases arising from triple negative breast cancer (see Part 8).

Although stage IV cancer is a very serious and incurable illness and has a worse prognosis than cancers caught prior to reaching this stage, women can enjoy a good quality of life after a diagnosis of metastatic cancer.

31. What is the difference between "local" and "systemic" therapy? Do I need both?

Local treatments, such as surgery and radiation therapy, are used to remove, destroy, or control the cancer cells in a specific area. In the case of breast cancer, these treatments are designed to remove cancer in the breast and lymph nodes, and to prevent recurrence of cancer in those areas. Systemic treatments, such as chemotherapy, are used to destroy or control cancer cells that may have escaped to other parts of the body and/or to prevent recurrence of cancer in parts of the body outside of the breast and local lymph node areas. Depending on the stage the cancer has reached upon detection, a patient may have just one form of treatment or a combination. Different forms of treatment may be given at the same time or one after the other. Talk to your doctor about the optimal order for your particular case.

32. Before I proceed with surgery and/or systemic therapies, how do I know that my breast cancer has not spread to other areas of my body?

It is not uncommon to worry that your breast cancer has spread from your breast to other parts of your body. In general, for patients with stage I and II triple negative breast cancers, a chest X-ray and routine blood tests (to include liver and bone enzymes) will be evaluated before you start your treatments. In the case of stage III triple negative breast cancer, your doctor will likely order more extensive radiological testing to ensure your breast cancer has not spread to organs outside of your breast. These tests would likely include a CT to include your chest, abdomen, and pelvis and a bone scan to assess for signs of metastases in your bones. If you are found to have radiographic evidence of metastases on either of these two scans, your doctor will likely order (assuming it is in a safe location) a biopsy to prove (or disprove) metastatic, or stage IV, disease.

SURGICAL TREATMENT

33. What is a mastectomy and how does it differ from a lumpectomy?

A mastectomy involves surgical resection of the breast. There are different kinds of mastectomies based on the amount of neighboring tissue, in addition to the breast, removed at the time of surgery. A **total (simple) mastectomy** involves removal of the whole breast, but does not involve removal of all lymph nodes under the arm. A **modified radical mastectomy** involves removal of the breast, the lymph nodes under the arm, and the lining over the chest muscles.

Total (simple) mastectomy

The surgeon removes the whole breast, but does not remove lymph nodes.

Modified radical mastectomy

The surgeon removes the breast, some lymph nodes under the arm, and the lining over the chest muscles.

Partial mastectomy

The surgeon removes the tumor, some of the normal breast tissue around it, and the lining over the chest muscles below the tumor.

Segmental mastectomy

Removal of the tumor, some of the normal breast tissue around it, and the lining over the chest muscles below the tumor.

In a lumpectomy, also called a **partial mastectomy**, only the tumor and a small section of normal breast tissue are removed from the breast, leaving the breast virtually intact. There is also a procedure that falls midway between a mastectomy and a lumpectomy called a **segmental mastectomy**. In a segmental mastectomy, the surgeon removes the tumor, some of the normal breast tissue around it, and the lining over the chest muscles below the tumor. Both lumpectomies and segmental mastectomies minimize the amount of breast tissue taken by the surgeon, and both should be followed by a course of radiation treatment; these therapies are referred to as "breast-conserving therapies" because the goal is to both remove the cancer and maintain as much of the original breast tissue as possible.

34. Which type of surgery is best for me?

Both forms of treatment, mastectomy and breast-conserving therapy, have their advantages and disadvantages. The goal of surgery is to physically remove all cancer cells from the breast and from lymph nodes under the arm. When tumors are very large or have extremely irregular shapes, modified radical mastectomies are more effective in achieving this goal than lumpectomies. However, there are drawbacks to totally removing the breast: In addition to the strain of major surgery on the patient's physical and emotional well-being, the loss of a breast can bring feelings of depression and insecurity and can inhibit the patient's sexuality. In cases in which it is medically appropriate, breast-conserving therapy can alleviate some of these potential problems.

Breast-conserving therapy has proven highly effective for smaller or more regularly shaped tumors that have not metastasized, and it is particularly attractive for women who want to preserve their breast as much as possible. Because only a small amount of breast tissue beyond the tumor is taken, radiation therapy is necessary to make sure that any remaining cancer cells are killed; these treatments can require daily (Monday through Friday) outpatient visits for as many as 6 weeks, with regular additional checkups afterward. Breast-conserving therapy is therefore a more extended course of treatment than mastectomy. It is also important to know that studies show women, who are appropriate for breast-conserving therapy, who elect mastectomy or breast-conserving therapy experience similar survival.

Your doctors will need to know whether your breast cancer has spread to neighboring lymph nodes, namely in the axilla (under the arm). Often, the surgeon will perform a **sentinel node biopsy**, in which a dye and/or radioactive particles are added to the area of the tumor to help locate the first lymph node draining the cancerous zone. The lymph node that is stained by the dye first is removed during surgery so the pathologist can look for breast cancer cells within it. If cancerous cells are present, the surgeon will likely perform a procedure called **axillary lymph node dissection**. This procedure involves removal of lymph nodes in the axilla; again, the nodes are then examined by a pathologist to determine whether cancerous cells are present. The presence or absence of cancerous cells in your axillary lymph nodes will help guide the treatment recommendations to most effectively treat your breast cancer.

In summary, the breast surgery that is best for you depends on the stage of your tumor and, to a certain degree, upon your personal preferences and priorities. If you are greatly concerned about how your body will look following surgery, you should discuss this with your doctor so she or he will know that this is a consideration in

Sentinel node biopsy

The addition of dye during breast surgery to help locate the first lymph node attached to the cancerous zone; the node is removed to prevent spread of cancer and biopsied to determine whether cancerous cells are present.

Axillary lymph node dissection

Removal of lymph nodes in the armpit during the initial surgery; the nodes are then examined by a pathologist to determine if cancerous cells are present.

choosing the type of surgery. Your doctor should be able to give you a detailed description of how your body will look following surgery and assist you in determining how to obtain a satisfactory result. Breast-conserving therapy may not be an option for you, but even if that is the case, there are still ways in which your surgeon could assist in restoring your physical shape through reconstructive surgery, either during or following the mastectomy, which will be discussed later in this section.

35. How should I prepare for my breast surgery and how long will it take me to recover?

Cancer surgery is performed by either a general surgeon or a surgical oncologist, a specialist trained in surgical removal of cancerous tumors. Prior to the surgery, you will meet your surgeon to talk about the procedure, ask any questions, and address any concerns you may have, particularly regarding possible side effects of the surgery, risks, and postsurgical care. In turn, your surgeon will ask whether you are taking any medications and will go over your medical records with you to make sure you are not on medicines that could affect the surgery. After you have discussed these details with your surgeon, you will sign a consent form that says the doctor can perform the surgery.

The hospital where your surgery is to be performed should contact you a day or so before the scheduled admission date to tell you what you should bring with you—clothing, medical records, insurance documents, and the like—and whether you should eat prior to coming to the hospital. If they don't contact you, call the hospital's information line; it is important that you are properly prepared for the surgery.

If at any time prior to the surgery you are unclear about what you need to do, what the risks are, or what is going to happen, be sure to ask. If you have trouble understanding the surgeon's answers or if you find that you are still nervous or frightened, ask whether one of the nursing staff can explain matters to you. A nurse may be able to simplify the process so that you can better understand it. Alternatively, some hospitals have a staff counselor or patient advocate who can help you to make sense of what you are about to undertake. Sometimes a visit to a counselor or chaplain can help you to work through your fears prior to surgery, and entering the process in a positive frame of mind will make the procedure and recovery seem easier. The ultimate point, however, is this: You might find the hospital and the surgeon intimidating or frightening, but the surgeon and staff are there to care for your health, both physical and emotional. You are the one with cancer and the one who is having the operation, so you have every right to ask questions, even if you feel foolish or are afraid to do so—but the hospital staff can't help you if you don't tell them you need assistance.

The time you will spend in the hospital recovering will vary depending on factors such as your overall health and the type of surgery you need. At most institutions, breast-conserving therapy is done on an outpatient basis, and only mastectomy patients are admitted overnight. Thus, many women are able to return home within a day of the surgery, but others require 2 or 3 days of hospital care. Return to normal activities, such as work and household chores, should wait for about 3 to 4 weeks to allow your body time to heal. Talk to your surgeon about your specific recommendations.

During surgery, your surgeon may place drains in the wound area to collect fluid that accumulates in the area

You are the one with cancer and the one who is having the operation, so you have every right to ask questions.

of the surgery. These drains usually consist of plastic tubing and suction bottles; the tube runs from under the incision to a bottle outside your body. These bottles will need to be emptied regularly—your doctor will tell you how often—and the fluid measured, and the place where the tube enters the skin must also be cleaned and covered with fresh dressings. You and your caregivers will be given training in these tasks before the surgery, and you should also be provided with written instructions. If you aren't, ask for them; don't rely on your memory. The drains will be removed when the fluid accumulation decreases—usually about 10 days after surgery. Removal is a quick, relatively painless procedure that does not require anesthesia or a hospital stay. At this point, your surgeon will give you arm and shoulder exercises and additional instructions to help you avoid the complication of **lymphedema** (see Question 37). Ultimately, the time required for recovery from surgery depends on the extent of the surgery, your overall health, and any complications that might arise.

36. Based on the extent of the breast cancer within my breast, I'm not a candidate for a lumpectomy. If I have a mastectomy, is it possible to reconstruct my breast?

In past decades, women who had mastectomies either did not undergo **reconstructive surgery** or had their reconstruction done at some time after the initial mastectomy. Current practices, however, have moved toward a far less radical approach: Surgeons generally attempt to ensure complete removal of the disease while sparing as much original breast tissue as possible. When breast-sparing procedures aren't possible, it has become quite common, indeed standard, to perform the reconstruction immediately following the mastectomy, for the simple reason that the psychological benefits are significant.

Lymphedema

A condition in which lymph fluid collects in tissues following removal or damage to lymph nodes during surgery, causing the limb or area of the body affected to swell.

Reconstructive surgery

The use of surgery to restore the form of the breast.

Waking up to a reconstructed breast is considerably less emotionally painful than dealing with the loss, however short term, of a part of one's body.

Immediate reconstruction can decrease the need for multiple operations, and results tend to be cosmetically superior to delayed reconstruction. However, certain clinical circumstances make delays preferable: If there's a chance radiation therapy might be necessary, the patient and the doctor should confer as to whether to wait, since some kinds of reconstruction involving implants are less successful when the patient subsequently undergoes radiation therapy. Also, the condition of the skin covering the site of the mastectomy is an important consideration; where there is a possibility of necrosis—particularly in women who smoke, are diabetic, or have a collagen vascular disease—the uncertainty of the skin's response to surgery could make it wiser to wait for some healing to take place prior to reconstruction.

Immediate reconstruction

Breast reconstruction at the time of oncologic breast surgery (i.e., mastectomy).

If reconstruction is something you would like to consider, you should discuss these factors with your treatment team before surgery so they can assess whether immediate reconstruction is a good option for you. If you can't decide whether you'd like reconstruction, or what kind of reconstruction you want, you are probably better off waiting and undergoing **delayed reconstruction**; your reconstruction can always be performed at a future date with just as successful an outcome.

Delayed reconstruction

Breast reconstruction that is performed months after initial breast surgery.

There are a number of options for reconstruction, and the type of reconstruction recommended by the surgeon will depend upon specific factors that affect each patient. For more information on different types of reconstructive surgeries and options, please see the resources listed in the appendix.

37. What is lymphedema and how should it be treated?

Lymphedema (properly called secondary lymphedema to distinguish it from the rare form some people are born with) is a condition in which lymph fluid collects in tissues following removal of, or damage to, lymphatic vessels during surgery, causing the limb or area of the body affected to swell. Left untreated, the swelling can interfere with healing of wounds and perhaps result in an infection; therefore, it is important to watch for signs of lymphedema—and not just immediately following your surgery. Lymphedema can occur weeks, months, or even years later. Lymphedema that appears long after cancer treatment ends can sometimes signal a recurrence of the tumor, and should be reported to your doctor. Lymphedema usually occurs in the hand and arm on the side of the breast surgery. Fluid accumulates in fatty tissues just below the skin, causing the limb to become swollen and stiff. The symptoms of lymphedema include a full or tight feeling in the limb or skin; decreased flexibility in joints, particularly hands and wrists; difficulty fitting into clothing, especially if this occurs in one specific area; and persistent swelling.

Acute lymphedema

A temporary condition that lasts less than 6 months in which the skin indents when touched and stays indented, but remains soft to the touch.

There are different types of lymphedema. **Acute lymphedema** is a temporary condition that lasts less than 6 months. The skin indents when touched and stays indented, but remains soft to the touch. The mildest form generally occurs within days after the surgery, and although it is uncomfortable, it is usually not painful. This type of lymphedema is often resolved within 1 week by elevating the affected limb or by working the muscle or muscles associated with it. A more severe form of acute lymphedema occurs 4 to 6 weeks following surgery and is considerably more painful because the lymph vessels themselves are swelling. Again, the most common form of treatment is to elevate the affected limb; in addition, your doctor will probably prescribe anti-inflammatory medications to ease the swelling in the lymph vessels.

Chronic lymphedema (lymphedema that lasts longer than 6 months) occurs when the damaged lymphatic system is not able to handle the increased flow of lymph fluid. A number of factors can contribute to the development of this problem, including the following:

Chronic lymphedema
Lymphedema that lasts for longer than 6 months.

- Radiation therapy or surgery
- Lack of preventive measures after surgery
- Infection and/or injury of the lymphatic vessels
- Lack of movement of the arm
- Medical conditions such as diabetes, kidney problems, high blood pressure, congestive heart failure, or liver disease
- Tumor recurrence or growth in an area of lymph nodes
- Cancer or cancer treatments that cause loss of appetite, nausea, vomiting, depression, anxiety, or problems with metabolism

Some factors listed here have more scientific evidence behind them than others, but whatever factors might cause it, chronic lymphedema is a serious condition that can be difficult to treat. Most episodes of lymphedema, whether acute or chronic, are treated through mechanical means (through elevation of the affected part, massage, or use of fitted clothing to keep even pressure on the edema) in collaboration with a physical or occupational therapist. Occasionally, these measures are complemented with antibiotics to prevent or eliminate infections. It is important for you to look out for signs and symptoms of lymphedema and bring these to your doctor's attention. It is also important to talk to your doctor about ways to prevent lymphedema, including avoidance of infection, blood draws, and blood pressure measurements of your affected arm after surgery; maintaining a healthy body weight and good nutrition; and wearing a compression sleeve on the affected arm while traveling on airplanes. See **Table 1**, adapted from the National Cancer Institute's Cancer-Net Service (http://cancer.gov).

RADATION TREATMENT

38. What is radiation therapy?

Radiation therapy
(also called
Radiotherapy)

Use of high-energy X-rays to kill cancer cells and shrink tumors.

External (beam)
radiation therapy

The X-rays come from radioactive material outside the body and are directed at the breast by a machine.

Radiation therapy (also called **radiotherapy**) is the use of high-energy X-rays to damage cancer cells and stop them from growing. Although there are a number of different procedures in development and in use to deliver radiation to the cancer zone, most patients receive **external radiation therapy**, in which the X-rays are directed at the breast by a machine. Radiation is very carefully targeted to affect a limited number of cells—any remaining cancerous cells and a very small portion of the normal cells surrounding them—in order to limit damage to normal tissues. The goal is to kill the diseased tissue while sparing healthy tissue, so the doctors in charge of your treatment will take numerous steps to make sure only the cancer zone is affected.

Radiation
oncologist

A cancer specialist who determines the amount of radiotherapy required.

Treatment with radiation therapy is supervised by a **radiation oncologist**, who determines the dose of radiation based on the size and shape of the breast and the location of the cancer. Radiation therapy is also used after surgery to eliminate any microscopic cancerous cells that might remain. Post-surgical treatment usually begins about 2 to 3 weeks following surgery. If chemotherapy has been prescribed, radiation therapy is

Table 1   Patient Teaching Guide for Preventing Lymphedema

1. Keep the arm or leg raised above the level of the heart, when possible. Avoid making rapid circles with the arm or leg to keep blood from collecting in the outer parts of the limb.

2. Clean the skin of the arm or leg daily and moisten with lotion.

3. Avoid injury and infection of the arm or leg:

   Arms
   - Use an electric razor for shaving.
   - Wear gardening and cooking gloves; use thimbles for sewing.
   - Take care of nails; do not cut cuticles.

   Legs
   - Keep the feet covered when going in the ocean.
   - Keep the feet clean and dry; wear cotton socks.
   - Cut toenails straight across; see a podiatrist.

   Either arms or legs
   - Use sunscreen.
   - Clean cuts with soap and water, then use antibacterial ointment.
   - Use gauze wrapping instead of tape.
   - Talk to the doctor about any rashes.
   - Avoid needle sticks of any type in the affected arm or leg.
   - Avoid extreme hot or cold, such as ice packs or heating pads.
   - Do not overwork the affected arm or leg.

4. Do not put too much pressure on the arm or leg.
   - Do not cross legs while sitting.
   - Wear loose jewelry.
   - Wear clothes without tight bands.
   - Carry a handbag on the unaffected arm.
   - Do not use blood pressure cuffs on the affected arm.
   - Do not use elastic bandages or stockings with tight bands.
   - Do not sit in one position for more than 30 minutes.

5. Watch for signs of infection, such as redness, pain, heat, swelling, or fever. Call your doctor immediately if any of these signs appear.

6. Do exercises regularly to improve drainage.

7. Keep regular follow-up appointments with the doctor.

8. Check all areas of the arms and legs every day for signs of problems. Measure around the arm or leg periodically, or if the limb seems swollen, use a tape measure at two consistent places on the arm or leg. Tell your doctor if the limb suddenly gets larger.

9. The arm or leg may be less sensitive. Use the unaffected limb to test temperatures for bath water or cooking.

10. Eat a well-balanced diet.

Treatment for Early-Stage Triple Negative Breast Cancer

generally given after chemotherapy. In some cases, however, radiation may be given prior to the chemotherapy or in conjunction with it. The decision depends upon the individual's situation.

For external radiation therapy, patients usually go to the hospital or clinic each day, 5 days a week for 5 to 6 weeks. If breast-sparing surgery was used, this treatment will be given to the whole breast. At the end of the treatment time, an extra boost of radiation that focuses solely upon the place where the tumor was removed is often given.

It is important to note that in the case of external-beam radiation, you will not become radioactive; nor will you pose a threat to those around you. The radioactive energy entering your cells cannot be re-emitted from your body to harm other people's cells. Don't be afraid to hug, kiss, or touch other people; you can't hurt them.

39. How should I prepare for radiation therapy, and what side effects should I expect?

Your treatment will be supervised by your radiation oncologist, who in turn has a team of people to help with the treatment sessions: a **radiation physicist**, who makes sure that the equipment is working properly and that the machines deliver the precise dose of radiation; a **dosimetrist**, who works with the oncologist and the radiation physicist to calculate the amount of radiation to be delivered; a **radiation therapist**, who positions you for your treatments and runs the equipment that delivers the radiation; and a **radiation nurse**, who coordinates your care, helps you learn about treatment, and tells you how to manage side effects. The nurse can also answer questions you or your family members may have about your treatment.

Radiation physicist

Makes sure that the equipment is working properly and that the machine delivers the right dose of radiation.

Dosimetrist

Works with the oncologist and the radiation physicist to calculate the amount of radiation to be delivered.

Radiation therapist

Positions patients for radiation treatments and runs the equipment that delivers the radiation.

Radiation nurse

Coordinates radiation therapy and patient care, helps patients learn about treatment, and assists in management of side effects.

Prior to beginning treatment, you will participate in a **simulation** (a planning session that allows the team to determine exactly where they want the radioactive beams to be applied). The doctors will review your medical history to determine where to focus the treatment, how much will be required, what type of radiation is required, and how many treatments you should have. They may also take CT scans to better locate the exact spot to be treated. Once the treatment site (also called a port or field) is determined, the radiation therapist will mark the target location or locations on your skin, usually with ink that may be permanent. Because the treatment requires you to lie absolutely still, the team may also create molds or immobilization devices to help prevent you from moving—particularly if the position of the cancer means you will be lying in an awkward or uncomfortable position during treatment. The simulation usually takes anywhere from 30 minutes to 2 hours, so be prepared for a lengthy session; actual treatment sessions are much shorter, about 1 to 5 minutes at most.

Simulation

A practice treatment that allows the radiation oncology team to determine exactly where they want the radioactive beams to be applied.

During the actual treatment sessions, you will be asked to change into a hospital gown so that the area to be treated can be exposed easily. The radiation therapist will position you on a table, place shields or blocks over you to protect healthy tissues and organs, and set up any devices created to help you stay completely still. Then the therapist will leave the room, although he or she will be able to see you and talk to you from the nearby room from which the radiation machines are operated. You should expect to see the machines in the room move around. They are being controlled from the next room by the radiation therapist.

The application of radiation takes only about 1 to 5 minutes, and you will feel, hear, see, and smell nothing—the treatment is entirely painless and is similar to having an X-ray. However, if at any time you feel uncomfortable or ill, you should immediately tell your radiation therapist; the treatment can be halted if necessary. Any other questions or concerns you may have about the session should also be directed to the radiation therapist.

Radiation treatment affects every patient differently, depending on the dosage and on the patient's overall health. That said, it typically causes only minor side effects, and some patients experience none at all. You will be given a list of likely side effects by your doctor or nurse. It's important to make sure that your doctor is aware of any medications you are taking, whether over-the-counter or prescription, or allergies you have so he or she can help you minimize side effects. Also, if you experience unusual symptoms, such as sweating, fever, or pain, tell your doctor immediately.

Most of the side effects related to radiation therapy are not serious, although they can be uncomfortable. Skin irritation, redness, itching, and similar symptoms are among the most common. These side effects are temporary, lasting about 6 weeks. Your radiation oncologist and treatment team will provide instructions for skin care during radiation to make your side effects more bearable. You may also have some minor, long-term changes, such as a darkening of the skin in the treated area and an increase in the size of pores in the skin. These changes can last a year or longer after treatment. There is also a condition in which small, red areas called **telangiectasias** appear. They are caused by dilation in blood vessels of the skin; these, too, should fade in time, although they can be permanent.

Telangiectasias
Small red areas appear on the skin, caused by dilation in blood vessels of the skin.

Some patients experience loss of appetite and difficulty in digestion during radiation therapy; it is not unusual for patients to lose several pounds during treatment. Fatigue is also fairly common, but it can be alleviated by taking a few simple steps. First, make sure you are getting proper nutrition. A second method of combating fatigue is, somewhat surprisingly, engaging in mild exercise. A short walk, for example, can sometimes reduce tiredness. If fatigue is severe or chronic, however, you might want to arrange to get assistance in everyday tasks, such as shopping or housework, to reduce the demands on your energy. Some patients go to their employers and request limited work hours or take time off during the weeks they expect to receive treatment. Fatigue can last 4 to 6 weeks after treatment ends, so it's important to pace yourself carefully. If you experience stiffness or difficulty moving the arm near your treated breast, ask your doctor for exercises to help alleviate the problem.

SYSTEMIC THERAPIES

40. What sort of things will my doctor be considering when selecting systemic treatments like chemotherapy to treat my triple negative breast cancer?

You will meet with your medical oncologist to discuss whether you would benefit from medicines to treat your breast cancer. As discussed earlier, triple negative breast cancer lacks expression of the estrogen receptor, progesterone receptor, and the HER2 protein. Thus, many common breast cancer therapies that block these receptors have not proven effective in the treatment of triple negative breast cancer. Medical oncologists rely heavily on chemotherapy to treat triple negative breast cancer. Chemotherapy is a drug that "poisons" rapidly

Medical oncologists rely heavily on chemotherapy to treat triple negative breast cancer.

dividing cells, both cancerous and noncancerous. Triple negative breast cancer cells divide very quickly, thus are good targets for chemotherapy.

The fact that your breast cancer is triple negative is an important consideration when your doctor decides on your systemic therapeutic plan. Other considerations will include the size and extent of your tumor, including whether your breast cancer has spread to the lymph nodes under your arm (axilla). It may seem obvious, but larger tumors are more aggressive; thus, chemotherapy is prescribed more commonly for larger tumors than for smaller tumors. In addition, breast cancer cells that have spread to the lymph nodes under the arm are more likely to spread to other parts of the body; thus, chemotherapy is generally recommended. Your overall physical health is also a very important consideration as your doctor develops your treatment plan. Your body must be strong enough to tolerate chemotherapy. Prior to prescribing chemotherapy, your doctor will review both your breast cancer history and your overall physical health in detail. And, finally, your personal feelings about chemotherapy are highly important as you and your doctor consider chemotherapy. It is important that you discuss any fears or concerns about chemotherapy before making final decisions about your treatment.

Many women find it helpful to talk to other women who have already completed chemotherapy to "demystify" the experience. The unknown is always difficult to face. Talking to other breast cancer survivors can be very helpful. You can find survivors through your doctor's recommendation, online resources, family friends, or the resource center within the medical center where you are being treated. Don't be afraid to ask!

41. I had my breast cancer removed and was treated with external beam radiation therapy. Isn't the breast cancer out of my body? Why would I need additional treatments like chemotherapy?

It is very common to wonder why chemotherapy may be necessary if your breast cancer has been surgically removed and/or your chest wall or remaining breast has been irradiated. At first glance, it appears that your breast cancer is essentially gone. Although your breast cancer is no longer able to be seen by the "naked eye," more than likely there are microscopic breast cancer cells left behind in the body. These small, microscopic breast cancer cells may find their home in organs outside the breast (i.e., liver, lungs, bones, lymph nodes) and grow such that your breast cancer may come back as metastatic. Once breast cancer becomes metastatic, or stage IV, it is rarely curable. Although there are many drugs to treat metastatic breast cancer (discussed later in Part 8), your doctor would like to prevent metastasis from happening in the first place. To protect you from your breast cancer returning, your doctor may prescribe chemotherapy to kill any microscopic breast cancer cells that survived your surgery or radiation.

42. Which chemotherapies are most commonly prescribed to treat triple negative breast cancer that is confined to the breast and/or lymph nodes?

Although there are over a dozen chemotherapies to treat breast cancer, several main classes of chemotherapy are commonly used to treat operable triple negative breast cancer. These three drug classes include (1) anthracyclines, (2) alkylating agents, and (3) taxanes (see **Table 2**).

Table 2   Drugs Used in the Treatment of Breast Cancer

Drug Name Generic (Brand), Maker CHEMOTHERAPY	Actions/Common Side Effects* The treatment of cancer using specific chemical agents or drugs that are selectively destructive to malignant cells and tissues.
ALKYLATING AGENTS	**Alkylating agents are a group of chemotherapy drugs that target the DNA of cancer cells to prevent the cells from growing or reproducing. Alkylating agents attack cancer cells in all phases and disrupt their growth. These cells are then destroyed.**
Cyclophosphamide (Cytoxan) Bristol-Myers Squibb	Cyclophosphamide (Cytoxan) is a chemotherapy drug commonly used to treat breast cancer and other cancers. Cyclophosphamide first disrupts cancer cells, then destroys them. Cyclophosphamide is taken in tablets by mouth or intravenously (through the vein) over 30 to 60 minutes. **Side effects may include** decrease in blood cell counts with increased risk of infection; nausea, vomiting, diarrhea, and abdominal pain; decreased appetite; hair loss (reversible); bladder damage; fertility impairment; lung and hearing damage (with high doses); sores in mouth or on lips; and stopping of menstrual periods. **Less common side effects**: decreased platelet count (mild) with increased risk of bleeding, blood in urine, darkening of nail beds, acne, fatigue, fetal changes if patient becomes pregnant when taking cyclophosphamide. At high doses, can cause heart problems. Urinary system problems and some secondary cancers have been reported.
ANTHRACYCLINE ANTIBIOTICS	**Anthracyclines work by deforming the DNA structure of cancer cells and terminating their biological function. They disrupt the growth of cancer cells, which are then destroyed.**
Doxorubicin (Adriamycin) Pfizer	Doxorubicin (Adriamycin) is a type of antibiotic used specifically in the treatment of cancer. It interferes with the multiplication of cancer cells and slows or stops their growth and spread in the body. **Side effects may include** decreased white blood cell count with increased risk of infection, decreased platelet count with increased risk of bleeding, loss of appetite, darkening of nail beds and skin creases of hands, hair loss, damage to the skin if drug gets outside the veins, nausea, and vomiting. **Less common side effects**: sores in mouth or on lips, radiation recall skin changes, fetal abnormalities if taken while pregnant or if patient becomes pregnant while on this drug. Patients should be tested for heart problems before beginning doxorubicin and should be continuously monitored for developing problems during treatment.

Table 2 Drugs Used in the Treatment of Breast Cancer (Continued)

Drug Name Generic (Brand), Maker	Actions/Common Side Effects*
Epirubicin(Ellence) Pfizer	Epirubicin (Ellence) was approved by the FDA in 1999 to treat early-stage breast cancer after breast surgery (lumpectomy or mastectomy) in patients whose cancer has spread to the lymph nodes. Epirubicin helps reduce the likelihood that breast cancer will return and improves a patient's chances of survival. Epirubicin is given intravenously (through the vein) in combination with two other chemotherapy drugs, cyclophosphamide and fluorouracil. **Side effects may include** nausea, vomiting, diarrhea, inflammation of the mouth, hair loss, damage to the skin if drug gets outside the veins, and reduction in white blood cells. **Less common side effects**: There is a risk of irreversible damage to the heart muscle associated with the drug. For women who receive epirubicin as adjuvant therapy, there is a slight increased risk of treatment-related leukemia. Epirubicin may cause harm to the fetus if taken while pregnant.
ANTIMETABO-LITES	**Antimetabolites prevent cells from making DNA and RNA by interfering with the synthesis of nucleic acids, thus disrupting the growth of cancer cells.**
5-Fluorouracil (5-FU, Adrucil, Fluorouracil) multiple makers	5-fluorouracil (5-FU) is a drug that kills cancer cells by stopping their growth. It can also make it hard for cancer cells to fix damage. **Side effects may include** decreased white blood cell count with increased risk of infection, decreased platelet count with increased risk of bleeding, drowsiness or confusion, darkening of skin and nail beds, dry, flaky skin, nausea, vomiting, sores in mouth or on lips, thinning hair, diarrhea, brittle nails, and increased sensitivity to sun. **Less common side effects**: darkening and stiffening of vein used for giving the drug, decreased appetite, headache, weakness, and muscle aches. Cardiac symptoms are rare but are most likely in patients with ischemic heart disease.
Methotrexate (MTX, Amethopterin, Folex, Mexate) multiple makers	Methotrexate prevents cells from making DNA and RNA by interfering with the synthesis of nucleic acids, thus stopping the growth of cancer cells. **Side effects may include** nausea (high dose), vomiting (high dose), sores in mouth or on lips, diarrhea, increased risk of sunburn, radiation recall skin changes, and loss of appetite. **Less common side effects**: decreased white blood cell count with increased risk of infection, decreased platelet count with increased risk of bleeding, and kidney damage (high dose). Liver, lung, and nerve damage are sometimes seen with methotrexate use, but the adjuvant drug leucovorin offsets the worst side effects.
TAXANES	**Taxanes are powerful drugs that can stop cancer cells from repairing themselves and making new cells. Often used for treatment of cancers that have not responded to or have recurred after anthracycline therapy.**

(continued)

Table 2   Drugs Used in the Treatment of Breast Cancer (Continued)

Drug Name Generic (Brand), Maker	Actions/Common Side Effects*
Docetaxel (Taxotere) Sanofi-Aventis	The FDA has approved docetaxel to be used as a single agent over a wide range of doses for the treatment of locally advanced or metastatic breast cancer in patients who have received prior chemotherapy. Docetaxel is also approved in combination with doxorubicin and cyclophosphamide for the adjuvant treatment of patients with operable, node-positive breast cancer. Docetaxel inhibits the division of breast cancer cells by acting on the cell's internal skeleton. **Side effects may include** decreased white blood cell count with increased risk of infection, decreased platelet count with increased risk of bleeding, hair thinning or loss, diarrhea, loss of appetite, nausea, vomiting, rash, and numbness and tingling in hands and/or feet related to peripheral nerve irritation or damage. **Less common side effects:** sores in mouth or on lips, swelling of ankles or hands, increased weight due to fluid retention, fatigue, muscle aches, loss of nails, and redness or irritation of the palms of hands or soles of feet.
Paclitaxel (Taxol) Bristol-Myers Squibb	Paclitaxel (Taxol) was first approved by the FDA in 1992 to treat advanced (metastatic) breast cancer. In 1999, the FDA also approved paclitaxel to treat early-stage breast cancer in patients who have already received chemotherapy with the drug, doxorubicin. Paclitaxel is called a mitotic inhibitor because of its interference with cells during mitosis (cell division). **Side effects may include** decreased white blood cell count with increased risk of infection, fatigue, numbness and tingling in hands and/or feet related to peripheral nerve irritation or damage, muscle and bone aches for 3 days, hair loss, nausea, vomiting, mild diarrhea, and mild stomatitis. **Less common side effects:** allergic reaction, skin rash, flushing, increased heart rate, wheezing, and swelling of face. Transient heart problems such as bradycardia occur in 30% or less of patients and are usually not severe.
Paclitaxel protein-bound particles for injectable suspension, nanoparticle albumin-bound (nab) paclitaxel (Abraxane)Abraxis Oncology	The nab paclitaxel uses nanotechnology to put paclitaxel in bits of the protein albumin so it can enter the cancer cells more easily. It is used for the treatment of breast cancer that has come back after combination therapy. Higher doses of paclitaxel are given. **Side effects may include** decreased blood counts with increased risk of infection and bleeding, numbness and tingling of the hands and feet related to peripheral nerve irritation, hair loss, muscle and bone aches for 3 days, nausea, and vomiting. **Less common side effects:** fluid retention and changes in heart test (ECG).

Table 2   Drugs Used in the Treatment of Breast Cancer (Continued)

ADJUVENT THERAPY	A variety of drugs that complement the chemotherapy regimen.
Leucovorin	Leucovorin is a form of vitamin used to offset the side effects of methotrexate and/or enhance the action of 5-FU. Leucovorin has few side effects itself, but its use with 5-FU can sometimes exacerbate the side effects of that drug.
Pamidronate(Aredia) Novartis Zoledronic acid (Zometa)Novartis	Both drugs are used to alleviate hypercalcemia; zoledronic acid is a newer, more powerful agent. **Both drugs have similar side effects, which may include** fever lasting for a short time (24 to 48 hours after infusion), pain at place of injection, and irritation of the vein used for giving the drug. **Less common side effects:** nausea, constipation, anemia, and decreased appetite. Renal function should be monitored with use of zoledronic acid. Zoledronic acid can cause bone damage (osteonecrosis) in the jaw.
ANTIEMETICS (ANTI-NAUSEA)	**Drugs used to prevent nausea or vomiting. Antiemetics work by a wide range of mechanisms.**
SEROTONIN ANTAGONISTS	**Serotonin antagonists suppress serotonin activity in the brain to prevent triggering of the vomiting reflex.**
Granisetron hydrochloride (Kytril) Dolasetron mesylate (Anzemet) Ondansetron hydrochloride (Zofran) Palonestron (Aloxi)	
Substance P/neurokinin (NK_1) receptor antagonist Aprepitant (Emend) Merck	Substance P/NK_1 receptor antagonists block nausea and vomiting pathways. They are given with a serotonin antagonist and dexamethasone to prevent nausea and vomiting.

*Drug information has been drawn from *The Physicians' Desk Reference*, the FDA Web site, CancerSource.com, Drug Guide, and, in some cases, specific pharmaceutical companies' Web sites. Not all known side effects are listed here; consult with your doctor if you are experiencing side effects, whether they are listed here or not. Many of these medications also have interactions with other medications that produce symptoms not listed here.

Treatment for Early-Stage Triple Negative Breast Cancer

Your doctor will likely prescribe a combination of each of these drugs to treat your triple negative breast cancer. The duration of your chemotherapy could last anywhere from 8 weeks to 6 months. Common combinations include (1) adriamycin plus cyclophosphamide (AC) every 2 to 3 weeks for 4 cycles with/or without paclitaxel every 2 to 3 weeks for 4 cycles, (2) Taxotere/adriamycin/cyclophosphamide every 3 weeks for 6 cycles, (3) Taxotere/cyclophosphamide every 3 weeks for 4 cycles, and (4) adriamycin plus cyclophosphamide (AC) every 2 to 3 weeks for 4 cycles followed by paclitaxel every week for 12 weeks. Each of the chemotherapies, how they work, and common side effects are listed in the table. The individual chemotherapies listed here are administered intravenously. Your doctor and/or medical oncology team will meet with you prior to your first cycle of chemotherapy to discuss what to expect, what medications to take to prevent nausea (**antiemetics**), and when you should call with concerns. You will also meet with your doctor and/or medical oncology team prior to each cycle to check your blood counts, discuss how you tolerated your last cycle, plan how to make the next cycle more tolerable, and ensure you have recovered from side effects of treatment. It is very important to talk to your doctor about your side effects so he or she can help troubleshoot your next treatment.

Antiemetics

Anti-nausea medications.

43. My doctor has recommended chemotherapy to treat my triple negative breast cancer. I have heard dreadful stories about chemotherapy. What should I expect, and how will my life be affected during chemotherapy?

Although chemotherapy can be very beneficial in treating your breast cancer, it can also have many side effects.

Side effects specific to particular chemotherapies are listed in Table 2. There are many side effects that are common to chemotherapy in general, in varying degrees, including fatigue, nausea and/or vomiting, hair loss, mouth sores, changes in bowel habits, and risk of infection. Other more rare and serious side effects might include damage to your heart muscle, allergic reaction, and risk of leukemia in the future. Luckily, decades of research have improved the experience of chemotherapy with drugs focused on **supportive care**. Examples include drugs to prevent/treat nausea (antiemetics) and others that boost the immune system, specifically white blood cells, to prevent infection (growth factors). You will receive specific instructions on how to prevent chemotherapy-related symptoms from your doctor and your medical oncology team. Specific symptoms and prevention/treatment strategies will be reviewed in detail in the next question.

Supportive care

Treatments devoted specifically to symptoms related to cancer.

44. How can I prevent side effects related to chemotherapy? Will my doctor give me specific instructions?

Some of the more common side effects from chemotherapy include fatigue, nausea and/or vomiting, hair loss, risk of infection, and risk of allergic reaction. We will review the more common side effects and potential prevention or treatment strategies here.

Fatigue

Fatigue is one of the most common side effects of chemotherapy, as well as radiation therapy. It is a complicated side effect because there are many factors that contribute to feelings of tiredness. It can even occur spontaneously in the absence of either of these adjuvant therapies. Yet resting—which seems the obvious solution for fatigue—sometimes does more harm than good: Rest too much, and your energy level actually decreases. So how does one properly deal with fatigue?

Unlike most other symptoms, fatigue is the one side effect that often isn't treated medically but through adjustments in diet and lifestyle. The reason for this is simple: Fatigue is a symptom that comes and goes, that isn't predictable in onset or duration, and usually reflects the exertion of the body as it attempts to heal. Unlike nausea or hair loss, fatigue isn't a sign of bodily dysfunction except when it is related to low blood cell counts; it is a normal reaction to the strain of rebuilding damaged cells, healing injuries, and fighting off illness, all of which are going on during the time a patient is undergoing treatment. As you undergo treatment, all of the healing systems of your body are pushing ahead to heal the damage being done by both the cancer and the treatment. The fatigue you feel is your body's way of signaling that you need rest and good nutrition to support this effort. "Curing" fatigue through the use of stimulants would simply wear out the body more in the long term, leaving it more vulnerable to opportunistic infections. Thus, except where red blood cell counts have dropped—something your doctor will monitor throughout your treatment—fatigue is not a symptom to be treated with medication (or blood transfusions) but rather is a signal that you should find ways to "reassign" your body's energy stores.

Nausea/Vomiting

Nausea and vomiting is not a topic most people care to discuss, but it's something that cancer patients must learn to deal with. These symptoms occur in almost 50% of patients undergoing chemotherapy and radiation therapy for cancer. The best way to approach the problem is to understand it, and this means knowing how to classify the symptoms. The National Comprehensive Cancer Network publishes patient guidelines (see the appendix) that detail five different classes of nausea and vomiting: acute-onset, delayed-onset, anticipatory, breakthrough, and refractory. Acute-onset nausea and vomiting usually occurs a few minutes to several hours after the chemotherapy is given, with the worst episodes occurring 5 or 6 hours after treatment; the symptoms end within the first 24 hours. Delayed-onset vomiting develops more than 24 hours after chemotherapy is given. It occurs commonly with cisplatin, carboplatin, cyclophosphamide, and doxorubicin, but the timing and duration depend on the particular drug. Anticipatory nausea and vomiting is learned from previous experiences with chemotherapy. As the patient prepares for the next dose of chemotherapy, she anticipates that nausea and vomiting will occur as it did previously, which triggers the actual reflex. Breakthrough vomiting occurs despite treatment to prevent it and requires additional therapy, while refractory vomiting occurs after one or more chemotherapy treatments—essentially if the patient is no longer responding to anti-nausea treatments.

Depending on the type of symptoms involved, different drugs called antiemetics are usually prescribed. Some of the most common medicines to prevent and/or treat nausea are called serotonin antagonists. They act upon the centers in the brain that trigger feelings of nausea. Antiemetic drugs are usually taken before the chemotherapy is given and/or at specific times related to when you take your chemotherapy, so it is important to be aware of the timing of your next treatment. It is very important to tell your nurse or doctor if you have nausea and/or vomiting. The antiemetic regimen can be changed so that you do not get sick after the next cycle of chemotherapy.

Hair Loss

Not all chemotherapy causes complete hair loss. However, all of the commonly used regimens to treat early-stage breast cancer do cause complete hair loss. Talk to your doctor about your particular regimen. If hair loss is expected, it usually occurs about 10 to 14 days following your first dose of chemotherapy. It is best to get fitted for a wig while your own hair is in place. It generally grows back to a "short hair style" length by 3 months after chemotherapy. Most insurance policies cover wigs; check with yours.

Risk of Infection

Most chemotherapies will place you at increased risk for infection, particularly when your white blood cell count is low (**neutropenia**). The risk is usually greatest about 10 to 14 days after your treatment. If you feel chilled, overly warm, or generally not well (especially during the 10- to 14-day time period), take your temperature. Call your doctor, or your medical team, for a temperature above 100.5 degrees F. If you develop a fever during chemotherapy, you will need to notify your doctor and/or medical team immediately to have your blood drawn to check for infection and to check your blood cell counts. If your blood counts are low, antibiotics may be necessary. You may need to be admitted to the hospital to receive antibiotics through your vein.

While you are receiving chemotherapy, you can take several precautions to lower the risk of infection. At anytime, it is best to wash fresh fruits and vegetables thoroughly with soap and warm water, and peel them if possible. You should also avoid crowds where encountering a sick

Neutropenia

A condition of an abnormally low number of a particular type of white blood cell called a neutrophil. White blood cells (leukocytes) are the cells in the blood that play important roles in the body's immune system by fighting off infection.

person is more likely (e.g., daycare, nursing homes), and engage in regular hand washing. If going to the grocery store or anywhere you may use a cart or basket, it is wise to wipe the handle with an antibacterial wipe (most grocery stores/major department stores now provide these).

Although it is okay to have visitors during chemotherapy, be sure that your friends and family wash their hands well before spending time with you. Children especially! It is best to avoid medications given by rectum, such as anti-nausea medications and enemas, during the days of lowest blood counts (10–14 days after chemotherapy), as they may lead to infections.

To help your blood counts rise more quickly during chemotherapy, your doctor may prescribe a shot to help "boost" your immune system. These therapies are intended for patients who developed very low white blood cell counts or a prior infection during chemotherapy, or they may be given to speed up the interval in which chemotherapy may be given (i.e., every 2 weeks instead of every 3 weeks, often called "dose dense" chemotherapy). These growth factors (i.e., Neulasta, Neupogen) are usually given as an injection under the skin by the patient or a family member after training by a nurse. You may also opt to return to your doctor's office to receive this shot. Your doctor will know whether you are appropriate for this type of treatment.

Risk of Allergic Reaction

Some patients are actually allergic to chemotherapy (or the fluids in which the chemotherapy is mixed). A common example in the treatment of breast cancer is paclitaxel. If you are being prescribed a chemotherapeutic agent with a known risk of allergic reaction, your doctor will discuss this potential side effect with you.

You will likely receive medications prior to your chemotherapy (e.g., steroids, antihistamines) to help prevent an allergic reaction. Your nurses will also monitor you closely during your chemotherapy infusion to ensure you are not reacting to it. It is very important that you tell your nurse if you experience back pain, shortness of breath, sweating, anxiety, or a "sense of doom" during chemotherapy so that the infusion can be stopped or slowed down.

Although this list reviews some of the more common side effects of chemotherapy, there are many more, and many that are more specific to one chemotherapy than others. For example, in addition to allergic reaction, **peripheral neuropathy** (a tingling sensation in the fingers and toes that can become painful or interfere with daily functions) is a common side effect of taxanes, such as paclitaxel and Taxotere. Although the risk of **premature ovarian failure** (or early menopause) is present with any chemotherapy prescribed for women at a younger age, cyclophosphamide is a known culprit. It is important to discuss the potential side effect profile of the chemotherapies you will receive with your doctor, both to be fully informed and to be prepared so you can best cope with, prevent, and treat these side effects.

Peripheral neuropathy

A tingling sensation in the fingers and toes that can become painful or interfere with daily function.

Premature ovarian failure

Early menopause.

45. Many of my friends have been taking pills to either block or lower estrogen levels to treat their breast cancer. Why is my doctor not recommending this type of therapy for me?

Drugs such as tamoxifen or aromatase inhibitors are commonly used to treat women with a history of breast cancer that expresses the estrogen and/or progesterone receptors. These drugs, which are in pill form, work by either blocking the estrogen receptor (tamoxifen) or decreasing production of estrogen in a post-menopausal woman's body (aromatase inhibitors). Breast cancer cells that depend on estrogen to grow are deprived of their "fuel" in the face of these treatments, and ultimately stop growing and expire. As discussed above, triple negative breast cancer cells—by definition—do not express the estrogen and/or progesterone receptor, therefore their growth is not affected by drugs that block these receptors. Clinical studies also show that women with triple negative breast cancer do not benefit from drugs like tamoxifen and/or aromatase inhibitors, thus your doctor is unlikely to recommend this type of therapy as part of your treatment plan.

OTHER CONSIDERATIONS

46. My doctor has used the terms neoadjuvant and adjuvant in regard to chemotherapy. What do these terms mean?

Your doctor may decide to treat your breast cancer prior to breast surgery. This approach is called **neoadjuvant chemotherapy**. There are many reasons to choose this approach. One of the most common reasons is to shrink a large tumor to either preserve a woman's breast at surgery (breast-conserving therapy) or ensure that the surgical margins around the tumor are free of cancer cells (also called negative surgical margins). There are some situations where women who undergo neoadjuvant chemotherapy still need a mastectomy. It is important to talk to your doctor to understand your individualized recommendation.

Another reason to consider neoadjuvant chemotherapy is as part of a clinical trial (see Part 9 for more information about clinical trials). One way that researchers are trying to improve the prognosis for women with

Neoadjuvant chemotherapy

Adjuvant that is started before primary surgery.

breast cancer is to test new drugs and/or new combinations among women before they have their breast cancer surgery. This allows a direct measure of how well the treatment is working and may lead to much faster progress in developing better treatments for breast cancer. Studies have shown that giving neoadjuvant chemotherapy is generally a safe strategy and that "delaying" the surgery to allow time to give chemotherapy first does *not* increase the chance of cancer spread. Also, women who undergo neoadjuvant chemotherapy and who have complete disappearance of cancer in their breast (termed a **pathologic complete response**) tend to have better outcomes when compared to those who have residual cancer in the breast following chemotherapy. Giving chemotherapy prior to surgery may allow your doctor to have a better idea of how effective it is and what your prognosis may be. Especially for patients with triple negative breast cancer, there are many research studies open to test new treatments, given in combination with standard chemotherapy, and we would encourage you to talk to your doctor about whether such an option might be right for you.

Another and often more common approach is to give chemotherapy after definitive surgery (either mastectomy or breast-conserving surgery), called **adjuvant** therapy. In this scenario, you would start chemotherapy after completely healing from your prior breast surgery, ideally within a maximum of 12 weeks from your surgical date.

Pathologic complete response

Disappearance of cancer cells in an organ (i.e., breast) following neoadjuvant chemotherapy.

Adjuvant

Treatment given after surgery to increase the chance of a cure and to prevent the cancer from recurring.

47. I worked prior to my breast cancer diagnosis. Is it possible to work during chemotherapy and/or radiation therapy?

The decision to work during chemotherapy and/or radiation is a personal one that may vary by patient and by occupation. For many women who work (and enjoy their work), maintaining their normal routine can be a source of stability during an uncertain time. Many women enjoy the camaraderie of conversing with their colleagues and the fulfillment their job brings to their daily life. Having a job that is flexible is often one of the factors that steer women toward continuing to work (even on an abbreviated schedule) during their cancer-related therapies.

On the flip side, some women are quite distressed by the prospect of working during chemotherapy and/or radiation. Considerations that may make working during cancer treatments more difficult include long commutes, a stressful work environment, a physically demanding job, and/or family obligations that may make working outside the home *and* treatment for cancer too much to handle. It is important to weigh all the upsides and downsides of working during chemotherapy with yourself, your family, and your doctor. Remember that no decision is permanent and your feelings about working during chemotherapy and/or radiation may vary at different times during your course of therapy.

48. Are there alternative or herbal therapies for breast cancer, and do they work?

We may be most familiar with modern Western medicine, but many people are becoming increasingly aware of, and attracted to, alternative philosophies of patient care, particularly East and South Asian methods, homeopathic approaches, and naturopathic medical systems. Though some people are skeptical about the effectiveness of these treatment methodologies, some of the herbs and techniques used in alternative systems may have legitimate healing properties. Yet there are so many medicines and therapies touted as the next new

No decision is permanent and your feelings about working during chemotherapy and/or radiation may vary at different times during your course of therapy.

treatment for cancer, it's hard to know where to start. Everything from shark cartilage to green tea extract to vitamin C to melatonin has been suggested as having curative properties. For a cancer patient anxious to find an effective treatment—or even a way to deal with unpleasant side effects—the list can be bewildering, yet a recent study of cancer patients showed that as many as 80% were using or had tried such treatments in conjunction with their standard therapeutic regimens, in the hope of either enhancing the action of the regimen or reducing the side effects caused by it. Unfortunately, a large proportion of the patients in the study were taking these alternative therapies without informing their doctors and were experiencing side effects because the therapies interfered with or interacted with the action of chemotherapy drugs. For this reason, many physicians are wary of alternative medicines. Yet part of the problem is that doctors fail to ask whether their patients are using alternative therapies, and patients don't think to tell them. So the most important point to make in any discussion of alternative therapies is *make sure your doctor knows about them before you start using them.*

Traditional Asian medicine is attractive to many people because it emphasizes a whole-body approach to disease. From this perspective, disease is the product of improper balance or disturbances of vital energies that connect mind, body, spirit, and emotion. To treat such imbalances, traditional Asian medicine uses techniques including **acupuncture**, herbal medicine, massage, and qigong, a technique based on controlled breathing and meditation.

Acupuncture

A Chinese therapy involving the use of thin needles inserted into specific locations in the skin.

Homeopathic and naturopathic medicines are also examples of complete alternative medical systems.

Homeopathic medicine is an unconventional Western system that is based on the principle that "like cures like"—that is, the same substance that in large doses produces the symptoms of an illness, in very minute doses cures it. Naturopathic medicine views disease as a sign that the processes by which the body naturally heals itself are out of balance, and it emphasizes health restoration rather than disease treatment. Naturopathic physicians employ an array of healing practices, including diet and clinical nutrition, homeopathy, acupuncture, herbal medicine, hydrotherapy (the use of water in a range of temperatures and methods of application), spinal and soft-tissue manipulation, physical therapy, therapeutic counseling, and pharmacology.

The list of alternative and complementary treatments is too long to discuss in depth, but there are a few treatments that have been shown to be effective in treating cancer symptoms and side effects; these will be discussed next. For more information on treatments not discussed here, visit the Web site of the National Institutes of Health's National Center for Complementary and Alternative Medicine, which hosts a clearinghouse of information on various alternative treatments (see the appendix for this and others).

Acupuncture

There are some alternative therapies that have been shown to be effective against certain side effects, particularly nausea, fatigue, and pain. One of the best known is acupuncture, which is a Chinese therapy in use for over 2500 years involving the use of thin needles inserted into specific locations in the skin. In 1997, after studying the treatment at length, the National Institutes of Health concluded that acupuncture does provide substantial relief of nausea and vomiting associated with chemotherapy and that further research was necessary to determine whether it may have some benefits in treating pain associated with some forms of cancer therapy.

Acupuncture's effectiveness in controlling nausea has been well documented, and some insurance companies have even begun paying for acupuncture treatments. If you are interested in acupuncture as a therapy for nausea, consult with your doctor. He or she might have a list of approved practitioners in your area. If not, the American Academy of Medical Acupuncture (AAMA) keeps a list of accredited practitioners nationwide, as well as laws governing the practice for your state and information regarding how acupuncture should be used. Contact information for the AAMA can be found in the appendix.

Mind-Body-Spirit Techniques

There are any number of techniques that focus the power of the mind and the spirit upon the body to help cure disease, including meditation, guided imagery, and prayer. These come in innumerable forms and can't be listed here, but the type of mind-body-spirit method a person might use is a very personal choice in any case. Do they work? That depends on what you expect of them. Studies have shown that mind-body-spirit techniques do affect patients in very positive ways, primarily with respect to quality of life. They promote relaxation, a more positive outlook, and a general sense of well-being. All of these feelings can promote increased immune activity, faster recovery, and better overall physiological health—but they work best in conjunction with standard treatments such as chemotherapy and radiation therapy. Most doctors would encourage their patients to use these techniques as adjuvant, not primary, treatments of cancer.

Herbal Remedies and Supplements

A number of herbal and supplemental treatments are said to be effective for breast cancer, and still others are said to work on the side effects of standard treatment methods. Many of these treatments have long histories of use in traditional societies, and, indeed, herbal and traditional medicines are often the source of medicinal compounds used in modern pharmaceuticals. Unfortunately, relatively few of even the best-known herbal remedies have undergone scientific testing to demonstrate their effectiveness. That doesn't mean they don't work; the few studies of herbal remedies that have been done show that some really do have positive effects. The basic problem, however, is that very few people, even trained herbalists with a genuine, legitimate knowledge of various herbs' pharmacologic properties, understand the full effects of these substances on the body—and there is extremely limited knowledge among herbalists and medical doctors alike of what interactions they might have with standard therapies.

Worse still, ready availability of supplements allows patients to self-medicate with vitamins, supplements, and herbs they don't properly understand. Supplements currently are not regulated, or even reviewed, by the Food and Drug Administration (FDA), so there is no oversight of formulas used in different brands, the quantity of active ingredients, or the purity of those ingredients. In short, there's no guarantee that the bottle you buy from the health food store contains what you think it does. Even if you try to make your own medicines with fresh ingredients, you could get into trouble if you don't have training in the preparation and use of herbs. This is not knowledge you can get from skimming through a book or looking on the Web. The correct use of herbs is a very tricky business, and in some cases, if you use too much or take it improperly (for example, eating it raw when you should be making a tea or infusion from its leaves), you can make yourself extremely sick, particularly if you are already taking chemotherapy drugs. Remember, during cancer treatment, your normal body systems are under extreme strain, and you could—with the best of intentions—overstrain your body if you take a supplement or herb without knowing its interactions and effects. Never begin a course of medication, of any type, without first checking with your doctor.

If you regularly use herbal preparations to treat minor illnesses, you don't necessarily have to abandon the practice. As noted, they often do have beneficial effects. However, the stress of illness on your body is significant enough that you would be well advised to consult with your doctor, your pharmacist, and a trained herbalist before using herbal medicines in conjunction with standard therapies. To find a trained herbalist, talk to the herbal specialist in your natural foods store or visit a store specializing in homeopathic medicine.

PART SIX

Survivorship: Life After a Diagnosis of Triple Negative Breast Cancer

I've completed my chemotherapy for early stage triple negative breast cancer. What is next? How often should I expect to be seen by my medical team?

I am concerned about the impact my triple negative breast cancer and treatments have had on my family, particularly my children. What resources are available?

What options exist to preserve fertility for women with triple negative breast cancer? Are they safe?

More . . .

49. I've completed my chemotherapy for early stage triple negative breast cancer. What is next? How often should I expect to be seen by my medical team?

Once you've completed the active phase of treatment for triple negative breast cancer, you will enter into a surveillance mode of care. This means that you will continue to see your doctor and medical team on a regular basis. Based on the 2006 update of the "Breast Cancer Follow-Up and Management Guideline in the Adjuvant Setting," you will see your doctor every 3 to 6 months for the first 3 years after treatment completion, then every 6 to 12 months for years 4 and 5, then annually. Your doctor will counsel you about the signs or symptoms of recurrence including new breast lumps, bone pain, chest pain, abdominal pain, dyspnea, or persistent headaches. You will be counseled to perform monthly breast self-examination and will receive regular mammograms. The schedule of mammograms includes a first post-treatment mammogram no later than 1 year after the initial mammogram that led to your diagnosis, but no earlier than 6 months after finishing radiation therapy. Your doctor, including the radiologist reading your mammograms, will help set the schedule for subsequent mammograms for surveillance of abnormalities. In addition, yearly gynecologic examinations are recommended.

Many women wonder why their doctors are not ordering tests, including blood and radiology tests, on a regular basis after they complete therapy for triple negative breast cancer. Routine laboratory tests, including tumor markers and radiographs, including CT scans and bone scans, are not recommended if patients are doing well. Studies have not shown that ordering these tests in the absence of symptoms helps women live longer after a diagnosis of triple negative breast cancer. If anything, these tests may serve to heighten anxiety and lead to unnecessary biopsies. If you do develop certain symptoms, your doctor will order the most appropriate test for you to determine the cause of these symptoms, which may or may not be related to your diagnosis of breast cancer.

50. Now that I've completed my treatments (either surgery and/or radiation and/or chemotherapy), I would have expected to feel relieved. Why do I feel so lost and anxious?

Treatments, including chemotherapy, surgery, and/or radiation can be emotionally taxing. Although you may think you should feel elated to have completed therapy for triple negative breast cancer, the time just following treatment completion can be a period of anxiety and mixed feelings. For one thing, you may be simply worn out from all of the treatments you have just courageously endured. You may think that you are supposed to "bounce back" into your life prior to breast cancer. It may take weeks or months to feel energetic physically. If your fatigue persists for months on end, it will be important to communicate this to your doctor so he or she can evaluate you for common causes of fatigue, including anemia (low red blood cell counts), hypothyroidism, or even unrecognized depression. It may seem counterintuitive, but exercise can often boost your energy level. Talk to your doctor about exercise programs you may wish to engage in. Many cancer centers have organized exercise programs for patients who have just completed cancer therapies. This can provide a source of support and physical activity.

During active treatment, you were likely focused on getting through the next round of chemotherapy or the last week of radiation. It is very natural to feel a sense of loss (particularly of a routine) or anxiety toward the end of active treatment.

Emotionally, you may be surprised by your inability to enjoy the first few weeks to even months after you complete your triple negative breast cancer treatments. You have likely been involved in weekly visits (or even daily visits during radiation) to your doctor's offices. You have been actively engaged in treating your cancer through surgery, radiation, and/or chemotherapy. During this time, you might have focused on getting through the next round of chemotherapy or the last week of radiation. Facing your days without the routine of active treatment can be anxiety-producing and sometimes even scary. You may find that you have fears of breast cancer recurrence now that you finally have the time and energy to reflect on what having a breast cancer diagnosis means to you. You may also find it unnerving not to see your doctor every few weeks for a checkup. In addition, friends and family members may expect you to "bounce back to normal" and may not completely understand the feelings you are experiencing. Be assured that your feelings are quite normal. You can take comfort in the fact that your triple negative breast cancer was treated in a manner most appropriate for you. Over time, life will begin to return to normalcy and you will ease back into your pre-breast cancer routine. It is important to realize, however, that you may never view life in the same way that you did prior to your diagnosis of breast cancer. Embrace your new life and live it to its fullest!

51. Is it normal not to have mood swings at diagnosis or following therapy for triple negative breast cancer? Could there be a delay in this response?

Everyone's response to a breast cancer diagnosis is different, so there's really no such thing as a "normal" response. Yes, many patients do experience mood swings following a diagnosis or treatment for breast cancer, but others don't; it really depends on your ability to absorb and cope with the situation. Some people respond with denial—they try to ignore the changes, but it gets awfully hard to do that when you're in the midst of chemotherapy. Others get angry, wondering, "What did I do to deserve this?" The answer is obvious, when you think about it: You did nothing wrong. You don't deserve it, but it's not a question of what you do or don't deserve—it's something that just happened. Getting mad about it doesn't change a thing. You might feel many emotions, some right away, some a little bit later. At first, you might not feel anything. A feeling of numbness or emotional paralysis isn't uncommon, but if it persists beyond a short time—a week or two—you may want to talk to your doctor, nurse, social worker, or therapist.

The most important thing regarding your emotional response is that you deal with it appropriately. Don't ignore your emotions—bottling them up simply makes matters worse, and you could find yourself getting angry or upset in unexpected and unhealthy ways. You don't want to take your anger out on your children or your spouse. Doing so helps no one and hurts everyone, including you. Whatever feelings you have, get them out somehow, whether it is through writing in a journal or through talking—to your spouse, a friend, a relative, a minister, or a counselor. Support groups are invaluable in this respect because everyone there has been through, or is going through, what you are experiencing right now. They will not only understand perfectly what it's like, they may have excellent advice on how to cope.

52. Since my breast cancer diagnosis, I have had difficulty concentrating and my memory seems a little slow. I am used to feeling "in control." Why is this happening and will this improve over time?

In a word: stress. Poor concentration is a classic symptom of high levels of stress in anyone, breast cancer patient or not. It's perfectly understandable too—you've just received shocking news and your world is turned upside down. Poor ability to concentrate is somewhat normal under these circumstances.

There are numerous methods to address this problem. A classic way to relieve stress is exercise. It doesn't have to mean signing up for aerobics classes at the local gym; regular walks in the park will do, as the main point is to get your body moving, even if only a little bit. Exercise may be difficult for you, however, if you are suffering from severe fatigue or nausea associated with treatment. A less physically strenuous method is to make use of mental relaxation techniques, such as **meditation** and **guided imagery**. Many cancer centers offer classes or group sessions to teach relaxation and meditation techniques. If yours does not, ask your doctor or nurse for a referral to one that does, or check with the National Center for Complementary and Alternative Medicine at the National Institutes of Health to find links to locations offering such services. You don't necessarily have to attend a class, however; meditation can be done simply by concentrating your mind on an inanimate object and focusing on it to the exclusion of all else, clearing the mind of worries, fears, and the millions of inane thoughts that cross our minds each minute. Alternatively, you can meditate on spiritual or religious teachings, many of which are

Meditation

A mental technique that clears the mind and relaxes the body through concentration.

Guided imagery

A mind-body technique in which the patient visualizes and meditates upon images that encourage a positive immune response.

offered in books that provide a topic for each day. This may take a little bit of practice—don't be discouraged if you can't master it the first few days you try it. Another possibility is to use relaxation techniques that combine physical activity with meditation, such as yoga, tai chi, or qigong. Classes in these techniques are widely available and can often be found through your local YMCA or church, or simply by looking through the yellow pages.

Talk to your doctor about the difficulties you are having, too. There are some chemotherapy regimens and even supportive medications like steroids that can contribute to mental confusion. It may be that this is as much a pharmacologic problem as an emotional one. Although it might not mean changing the regimen, there could be ways of reducing the problem—altering the timing of your medication, for instance, so you take it later in the day or at night, leaving you better able to concentrate during your normal daily activities. You could also be suffering from depression, which can be treated. Finally, you may be experiencing problems with your sleep, either because of stress, hot flashes, medications, or other reasons. Addressing your sleep problems may also improve your concentration and mental clarity.

53. I've completed my breast cancer treatments but find myself thinking and/or worrying about it all of the time. How can I move on so my breast cancer won't rule my life?

It would be unrealistic to expect you to move on from your triple negative breast cancer diagnosis and treatment never to think about the experience again. **Perseverating**, or thinking about your breast cancer and its

Perseverating

Uncontrollable repetition of a thought, despite the absence of a stimulus.

potential return constantly, will more than certainly interfere with your daily activities, relationships, sleeping patterns, appetite, and ability to enjoy your daily life. You will likely be unable to tackle this situation on your own. If it arises, it will be important to talk to your doctor about your feelings so that you can get the most appropriate help. You may be dealing with **situational depression** or **anxiety** prompted by your breast cancer diagnosis that can be alleviated with appropriate counseling and/or pharmacologic therapies. Joining local support groups and/or connecting with other breast cancer survivors may also be helpful. Another often-successful strategy is to set aside time every day, even 15 to 30 minutes, to devote to thoughts surrounding your breast cancer diagnosis. Reserve this time to feel your emotions—for example, anger, fear, sadness—reserving the rest of the day for yourself, your family, your interests, etc., and knowing that you can always return to your thoughts the next day.

54. Why do I feel it is so hard to talk with my family and friends about my triple negative breast cancer diagnosis? I have a lot of guilt about the impact my diagnosis and treatment will have on my loved ones.

Cancer is difficult enough to accept when you hear the diagnosis from your doctor. Yet somehow, telling the people you care about is even more difficult. There are a number of reasons for this: First, telling people about the diagnosis makes it seem that much more "real" to you at a time when you might still be wishing that it wasn't real. Saying repeatedly, "I have breast cancer" to various family and friends effectively drills this fact into your mind—and who wouldn't prefer to pretend that this wasn't the case?

Situational depression or anxiety

Feelings of depression or anxiety that are prompted by a specific life event or situation.

Second, telling your friends and loved ones is painful because you have to see their reactions, which might mirror your own: shock, fear, and grief. Many newly diagnosed patients feel guilt at causing these emotions in people they love, which makes them all the more reluctant to tell their family and friends. There's also a certain level of fear that your loved ones, knowing you have cancer, may distance themselves from you. It hasn't been that long since cancer was instinctively identified as automatically terminal. You may also have practical concerns about job security—will you get fired or demoted if your boss believes your illness or treatment interferes with your productivity?

It might seem that hiding the truth is your best strategy, but be practical: It's physically impossible to keep the truth from those closest to you. You're going to have surgery, probably also a round of radiation and/or chemotherapy, and the effects of these treatments will be highly visible. Sooner or later, they'll know something is wrong—and if any of them have ever had a friend or relative with cancer (you'd be amazed at how many have seen it before), they'll quickly figure out what is going on. Hiding the truth will accomplish nothing positive and will do much damage to your relationships with your loved ones. Your friends and family may feel deceived and hurt, and you'll lose the goodwill of the people you most need to support you during your treatment.

For those closest to you—your spouse or partner, your parents, your siblings, your best friend—it's probably best to tell them yourself. For others who may be more distant, you may be able to enlist the assistance of a friend or relative to pass the news along. In reality, you will need to lean on the people closest to you as you embark on your treatment for triple negative breast cancer. Those you are closest to are the ones who are going to drive you to your doctor's appointments when you're feeling weak and nauseous, make your meals, pick up your medications from the pharmacy, and take your children to school when you're too fatigued to do it, and they're the ones you'll talk to when you need encouragement and companionship. Don't make their job any more difficult by not telling them what they need to know from the outset.

Patient comment:

I too feel a lot of guilt over having breast cancer twice and all that goes with it. The medical bills, the stress, the cancer wreaking havoc on your life, surgeries, illness, all the doctor and clinic visits, the life of your loved ones. It's not my fault, it's not my fault. Why won't it go away?

I try to change my way of thinking, but my guilt remains. Talking to my family has been a challenge. They do not understand TNBC, our fears, our worries that we cannot "do" anything except wait and see, trying to stay busy in our lives and not think about it. The problem is that we need to talk, to get it out. Many around us think we should just forget about it, it's gone. I wish. I find that online support groups help me with this problem, this release and supporting of others. Some loved ones may come to understand to the best of their ability. Others, their eyes glaze over. What is wrong with you, get over it! How can they understand, really?

55. I am concerned about the impact my triple negative breast cancer and treatments have had on my family, particularly my children. What resources are available?

Triple negative breast cancer isn't something that affects just you. It affects all the people in your life, including your spouse, your children, your extended family, and your friends. They may not have a good understanding of what triple negative breast cancer means, and like you, they have many different reactions—feelings of fear, anger, denial. They may find it hard to be supportive of you because they are struggling with their own emotions. Furthermore, they may find it difficult to give you the time and energy you are going to need. If your spouse works 14-hour days, for instance, he may not have the energy to drive you to your chemotherapy sessions. The key is to find ways to help your family to work with this difficult situation. That could mean using one of many strategies:

- Don't refuse offers of assistance. Members of your extended family, friends, or coworkers may offer their assistance. "If there's anything I can do to help, just let me know," is a common response when a friend is in need. It might be second nature to simply reply, "Thank you, but it's under control," yet this is your opportunity to obtain some relief for your family that you may not yet realize they are going to need. Break the habit of automatically refusing; make sure that anyone who makes this offer understands that you may need to take him or her up on it. For instance, have your friends, neighbors, and church members sign up to drive you and sit with you during your chemotherapy sessions. Even people you don't know very well may be willing to do things like help with yard work, take your car for an oil change or fill-up, and similar small but necessary tasks.
- Find ways to adjust the household routine so it doesn't overburden your family. You may not be able to do as much around the house if your treatment causes you to become tired and nauseous, but family

members picking up the slack may become tired and overstressed. Think about the tasks that must get done and find ways to minimize them. For instance, if you used to do all the grocery shopping, you might get a shopping service to do this instead of asking your partner to take on the additional task. House cleaning, laundry, and similar tasks can all be done by commercial services—some of which are specifically devoted to cancer patients at a minimal fee. Talk to the volunteers in your cancer center's resource center to find out what may be available in your area.

- Find assistance with child care. You don't have to hire a nanny just because you're sick. You might simply take advantage of school-based before- or after-school programs, or ask a relative or friend to pick the children up after school a few days a week. Some local YMCAs will pick up children at school and take them to a central facility where the kids can do homework and participate in activities for several hours. You may find that having the extra time helps you to balance the demands of your family and your illness better, and the costs associated with this program may be tax deductible.

- Consider a leave of absence from work—for either you or your spouse. Under the Family and Medical Leave Act, either you or your spouse may be able to take a 12-week unpaid leave of absence from your job, depending on whether your work situation qualifies. To determine whether one or both of you are eligible, check with the Department of Labor regarding the Family and Medical Leave Act.

- Take advantage of support programs for cancer patients. The American Cancer Society has a number of programs aimed at cancer patients in general and breast cancer patients specifically. The "Road to

Recovery" program, for instance, offers rides to treatment sessions, while the "I Can Cope" service provides a series of seminars on how you and your family can adjust to life with cancer. Other similar programs are widely available; ask your doctor for a referral or contact your local American Cancer Society chapter for more information.

56. Now that I have undergone treatments for breast cancer, my body seems very different. I don't feel as attractive. Will this feeling fade? What can I do to feel better?

Our culture has traditionally stressed breasts as a fundamental part of feminine beauty and sexuality, so losing one or both breasts or even scarring to the breast as a result of treatments for triple negative breast cancer can be traumatic. It's not unusual for women, even women who were confident about their attractiveness prior to their mastectomy, to feel insecure about their sexuality after losing a breast.

It's not unusual for women, even women who were confident about their attractiveness prior to their mastectomy, to feel insecure about their sexuality after losing a breast.

There are several ways to approach this problem. Breast reconstruction restores the shape of the breast, but cannot restore normal breast sensation. With time, the skin on the reconstructed breast becomes more sensitive, but it will never be the same as before a mastectomy. Breast reconstruction often makes women more comfortable with their bodies, however, and helps them feel more attractive. If you opted against reconstructing your breast initially (immediate reconstruction), but find that you've changed your mind, talk to your doctor— reconstruction is still a viable option. This approach is called delayed breast reconstruction.

Alternatively, you can approach the feelings of insecurity from the inside, through counseling. A therapist can help you to adjust and accept the changes that have occurred in your body, so that the loss of the breast doesn't affect your image of yourself as beautiful. Indeed, there are some women who adopt the stance that society's view of breasts as essential to feminine beauty is something they can reject by accepting their body as it is, with or without breasts.

These options work well when dealing with one's confidence strictly in the sense of public personal appearance. But what do you do when you have to show your body to your partner? In particular, the first occasion that your partner sees you after the surgery can be extremely uncomfortable. Moreover, the breasts and nipples are sources of sexual pleasure for many women. Touching the breasts is a common part of sexual intimacy in our culture. After a mastectomy, the whole breast is gone—it's not something you can hide or disguise. How do you deal with that?

It is important to address ways to mitigate the discomfort or embarrassment to make sure both you and your partner are prepared for what you are going to see and experience on the first viewing of your changed body. Talk about it beforehand as much as you need to—with a relationship or marriage counselor if you find that simple one-on-one discussion is too awkward at first— and continue to be open with your partner as you begin to reacquaint yourselves with the changes to your body. The first time you are intimate with your partner might bring on many difficult emotions or revive feelings you thought you were done with—anger, fear, "why me?"— so be prepared for what might be a difficult encounter. Remember that with time and compassion from each of you to one another, the discomfort will eventually pass and may bring you even closer together.

57. How do my partner and I "deal" with my breast surgery? How might I expect my diagnosis of triple negative breast cancer to affect intimacy and sexuality?

A mastectomy can greatly affect a woman's body image and feelings of attractiveness, but it certainly does not mean you will no longer have a sex life. Some women who have had a mastectomy feel self-conscious with greater visibility of their missing breast during intimate moments. It is important that you and your partner discuss what is and what isn't comfortable (both physically and emotionally) and ways in which to minimize your feelings of exposure.

If surgery removed only the tumor (segmental mastectomy or lumpectomy) and was followed by radiation therapy, the breast may still be scarred. It also may be different in shape or size. During the radiation period, the skin may become red and swollen. The breast also may be a little tender, but this should pass. Following healing, breast and nipple feeling should remain relatively normal.

Breast surgery or radiation to the breasts does not physically decrease a woman's sexual desire, nor does it affect her physiological responses during sex. Some good news from recent research is that most women with early-stage breast cancer have good emotional adjustment and sexual satisfaction by a year after their surgery. They report a quality of life similar to women who never had cancer. Whether you had a mastectomy or lumpectomy with radiation, communication between partners will be key to restoring and/or maintaining intimacy.

58. What strategies are available to help restore intimacy after treatment for triple negative breast cancer?

When you are in the midst of therapy (surgery, radiation, and/or chemotherapy) for your triple negative breast cancer, intimacy may be the farthest thing from your mind. You are dealing not only with the emotional upheaval of a new breast cancer diagnosis, but also with the physical side effects of therapy—which might include pain, nausea, vomiting, and/or fatigue. You have also just undergone therapies or are receiving treatments that have altered your body, which might include breast surgery or hair loss. Moreover, your already-full life now includes making trips to your doctor's office, coordinating child care, and off-loading household chores and/or work responsibilities. Feeling less sexy is normal.

Now that you may have completed your treatments, you may be wondering if your sex life is only a distant memory. It certainly does not have to be. You and your partner may feel closer than ever, as you have both banded together to face your breast cancer diagnosis and journey. As follows, you would like for your emotional closeness to also include physical closeness. Several challenges that may have been more prominent during therapy may seem less difficult. For instance, your energy level will likely be improving as your active therapy has ceased, making your ability to engage in intimate moments more feasible. You may be becoming more comfortable with your new body, and your hair is likely beginning to fill in. You may, however, have new challenges such as vaginal dryness—a result of premature menopause—and/or breast pain following surgical treatments and/or radiation. The use of non-estrogen-containing vaginal lubricants, which can decrease pain associated with intercourse, can help make your experience more enjoyable. If you are having significant difficulties with your body image and/or relationship following your treatments for triple negative breast cancer, it is important to bring this to your doctor's attention. You do not need to feel ashamed as these difficulties are very common and are usually easily resolved with appropriate one-on-one or marital counseling.

59. I have always wanted a family. Can I have children after a diagnosis of triple negative breast cancer? If so, when is it safe for women to become pregnant after a diagnosis of triple negative breast cancer?

It is not unusual for women who have had breast cancer to subsequently have children. This end result, however, requires foresight and careful planning in the choice of therapies and/or incorporation of fertility preservation strategies among young women being treated for triple negative breast cancer. The possibility of retaining your fertility and safely carrying a pregnancy depends in large part upon your diagnosis, the particulars of your tumor, and the treatment you receive.

A recent study showed no increase in cancer recurrences for women who became pregnant after breast cancer. For the few women who did have a recurrence, however, that recurrence happened faster if they became pregnant. Because pregnancy raises estrogen levels in the body, it is important for women to discuss their individual medical history and the safety of pregnancy with their doctors. Women are usually advised to wait 2 to 5 years (disease free) after the completion of treatment to become pregnant. (The first 5 years is the most likely time period for a recurrence.) Women should also discuss the impact of pregnancy on their general health, as chemotherapy can sometimes cause undetected damage to the heart and lungs.

Studies show that children born to cancer survivors after cancer treatment appear to have no more birth defects than children born to the general population.

Studies show that children born to cancer survivors after cancer treatment appear to have no more birth defects than children born to the general population. In addition, they have no greater risk for developing cancer, except in rare cases of truly genetic cancers.

In many women, cancer treatment causes menstruation to stop temporarily. This is a normal bodily response to a high degree of stress—a way of conserving bodily resources for the high-priority task of healing, rather than expending them unnecessarily on reproduction. Most of the time, menstrual cycles resume within a few months of the end of treatment, but there is no absolute guarantee that this will occur; you might find that your menstrual cycles come less frequently, that you sometimes skip one or more periods, or even that they don't come back at all. Both radiation and chemotherapy can affect fertility permanently, particularly if you are already older than 40 years of age and approaching the normal age for menopause. Some chemotherapy regimens can cause premature menopause, so if you had been considering having children prior to your cancer diagnosis, make sure your oncologist is aware of this fact before you undergo any sort of treatment. If your cancer is advanced enough to require very aggressive therapies (including chemotherapy and/or radiation), you might consider consulting with a fertility specialist before beginning your treatments. One option is to have ova extracted from your ovaries prior to treatment, fertilized in vitro, and frozen to await implantation after your treatment is done (see Question 61). This method allows you to potentially have a biological child even if your ovaries do shut down permanently because of the chemotherapy regimen you are on—but it can be extremely expensive, and is not always covered by insurance.

As noted earlier, many doctors suggest a waiting period of 2 to 5 years following treatment for breast cancer before you get pregnant. Because most signs of recurrence occur within this time, waiting allows you to be reasonably certain of your health prior to beginning a pregnancy. If you don't feel you can wait that long because of your age, you should discuss your wishes with your doctor. You will want to ensure that your body has completely recovered from the effects of treatment before subjecting it to the stresses of pregnancy.

If your future ability to breast-feed is important to you, bring up the subject to your surgeon and your oncologist before undergoing any treatment. Although they might not be able to do anything about it—after all, the top priority is ridding your body of the cancer, and breast-feeding is a secondary concern—if you let them know this is important to you, they'll do the best they can.

60. I've heard that chemotherapy can put women into early menopause. What breast cancer treatments put a woman's fertility at risk?

Chemotherapy presents the main risk to a patient's fertility. Triple negative breast cancer patients usually receive AC (adriamycin and cyclophosphamide), or less commonly CMF (cyclophosphamide, methotrexate, and 5-fluorouracil) chemotherapy. Cyclophosphamide (Cytoxan) is known to have a negative effect on ovarian function. Women receiving cyclophosphamide are four times more likely to develop ovarian failure, compared with controls. The chance of immediate ovarian failure increases with age. For CMF it is 78%, and for AC it is 38% (for a 40-year-old breast cancer patient). The risk of ovarian failure depends on a patient's age. For example, with AC chemotherapy, the risk of premature menopause is much lower in women younger than age 35 but nearly 100% in women age 50 or higher when they receive chemotherapy. Many triple negative breast cancer patients will also receive a taxane (either docetaxel or paclitaxel). Results of studies evaluating the additive risk of premature menopause when adding a taxane to cyclophosphamide-based chemotherapies have been mixed.

Radiation and surgery can also impact a patient's fertility if they affect the reproductive organs—namely the ovaries or uterus. This is not generally the case for most breast cancer patients. However, since each course of chemotherapy will result in the loss of a significant portion of ovarian reserve, even those who do not immediately become menopausal following chemotherapy are likely to experience early menopause. In addition, as previously noted, many experts do not recommend pregnancy for at least 2 to 5 years (recurrence free) after breast cancer diagnosis and treatment. During this interval, many patients who are not immediately infertile after chemotherapy will become infertile due to their diminished ovarian reserve and natural aging. Patients should work closely with their doctors to address these issues.

61. What options exist to preserve fertility for women with triple negative breast cancer? Are they safe?

Several treatments are available for women facing treatments for breast cancer, including the triple negative subset, to preserve their fertility. The availability and efficacy of these treatments vary based on a number of biomedical and social factors. Some of these options are well-established, while others are experimental. Factors such as cost, partner status, the patient's age, and diagnosis may influence the choice of an option. An excellent resource that reviews fertility preservation options for women being treated for cancer, including financial concerns, is Fertile Hope (http://www.fertilehope.org; see the appendix).

Options for preserving fertility include the following:

- *Embryo freezing* is the most established method of preserving a woman's fertility. Hormones are used to mature a woman's eggs, which are then removed and fertilized by in vitro fertilization (IVF). Embryos are then frozen for future use. This process requires sperm provided by a husband or partner. Donor sperm can also be used. All of the steps required to freeze embryos take about 2 to 6 weeks, depending on the type of stimulation used. Many centers require that the patient's breast tumor be surgically removed prior to embryo freezing, as the hormones used to mature the eggs may fuel the growth of the breast tumor.
- *Egg freezing* is an experimental option that may be attractive to single women who do not have a male partner and do not want to use donor sperm. Although egg freezing pregnancy rates are lower than embryo freezing pregnancy rates, the techniques are improving rapidly. For the woman, the steps required to freeze eggs are the same as those required to freeze embryos, and they take about 2 to 6 weeks.
- *Ovarian tissue freezing* may be a good option when there is little or no time for ovarian stimulation before treatment. Tissue from the ovary is removed,

cryopreserved (frozen), and then re-implanted later. Ovarian tissue freezing is still experimental. Some tissue transplants have been successful and have caused women to resume hormonal functioning, but (as of 2005) there have been only two live births to date.

- *Gonadotropin-releasing hormone analog (GnRH-a) treatment* is an experimental treatment that is sometimes offered during chemotherapy treatment. It is thought to protect ovarian function by temporarily putting the ovaries into a dormant state. Results of studies have been mixed, and more research is needed to determine whether GnRH-a treatment is safe and effective. Some fertility preservation options such as embryo freezing and egg freezing require hormone stimulation. The hormones used can raise a woman's estrogen level, which can be a concern for breast cancer patients, especially those with estrogen receptor-positive tumors. There are, however, some techniques that can be used, such as tamoxifen-IVF or letrozole stimulation, which may be safer for breast cancer patients. In addition, many oncologists feel that one round of stimulation before chemotherapy is acceptable. Patients need to discuss these risks and benefits with their doctor to understand which option is safe for them.

62. My doctor has ordered a bone mineral density test to determine if I developed bone loss during chemotherapy. What can I do to help build bone strength following treatments for triple negative breast cancer?

Your bone health can easily be evaluated with a series of X-rays called a bone mineral density test or DEXA (dual energy X-ray absorptiometry) scan. Your doctor will receive a score of your bone health that will tell you if your bone density is normal, osteopenic (weak), or osteoporotic (weak to the point that you might develop a fracture).

It is recommended that all women over the age of 50 years undergo routine DEXA scans under the direction of their general physician (i.e., internist or family practitioner). Your medical oncologist may recommend you undergo a DEXA scan even prior to the age of 50 years due to the effects of chemotherapy on your body. For instance, premature menopause, as a result of chemotherapy, makes women more prone to osteopenia and/or osteoporosis.

One study shows that younger, premenopausal women treated with chemotherapy experience bone loss during chemotherapy regardless of whether their menses stops. Interestingly, administering a bisphosphonate (a medication used to treat osteoporosis) prevented this bone loss. Moreover, a study conducted in Europe showed that women with estrogen receptor-positive breast cancer who received a bisphosphonate had lower rates of breast cancer recurrence, compared to those who did not receive this treatment. Whether this strategy is as beneficial in triple negative breast cancer patients is not yet known. This question is the focus of a large trial being conducted in the United States.

In the meantime, it is important to discuss the effects of your treatments on your bone health with your doctor so you can decide on the best treatment and surveillance strategy. In addition, consuming approximately 1200 mg of calcium and 800–1000 international units of vitamin D daily, and engaging in regular weight-bearing exercises (including walking and/or running) can help maintain and/or improve your bone health.

63. In addition to calcium, my doctor has recommended I take vitamin D supplementation. Is this for my bones, my breast cancer, or both?

Recently, vitamin D has become a focus among breast cancer researchers. Vitamin D has many health-related benefits including the promotion of bone health, immunity, and even cardiovascular health. Research studies have indicated that close to 75% of women with early-stage breast cancer have either insufficient or deficient levels of circulating vitamin D. More importantly, and when looking back at breast cancer outcomes for women with sufficient, insufficient, or even deficient levels of vitamin D, those with sufficient vitamin D values fared better.

Your doctor may check your vitamin D levels through a blood test sometime during the course of your breast cancer treatment. If your levels are sufficient, you will likely be encouraged to consume calcium and vitamin D to maintain your bone health. If levels are insufficient or even deficient, your doctor may prescribe higher levels of vitamin D for several months to boost your values to protect your bones and hopefully improve your breast cancer outcomes.

64. Is it true that there is a link between breast cancer recurrence and drinking alcohol?

Excessive alcohol intake is known to negatively affect health in a variety of ways. A recent study also indicates that higher amounts of alcohol intake may be linked to a higher risk of breast cancer recurrence. Women diagnosed with breast cancer between 1997 and 2000 were enrolled in this study on average 2 years after their original breast cancer diagnosis. They were asked about their alcohol consumption over the past 12 months, including how often and how much alcohol they drank. After following these women for an average of 8 years, this study found that alcohol was associated with a 30% increased risk of breast cancer recurrence among women who drank at least half a drink or more per day, compared to women who didn't drink at all.

Although these results need to be validated in other studies and this study was not specific to triple negative breast cancer patients, consuming more than a moderate amount of alcohol appears to be inadvisable from both a breast cancer standpoint and an overall health standpoint.

65. In addition to surgery, radiation, and/or chemotherapy, what can I do to keep my body healthy after a diagnosis of triple negative breast cancer?

In addition to regular visits to see your doctor and keeping up with your breast imaging and surveillance, you may be wondering what other strategies you can engage in to keep your body healthy following a diagnosis of triple negative breast cancer. One of the most important things you can do to maintain your physical health is engage in a regular exercise program and consume a balanced diet full of fruits and vegetables. By doing so, you will maintain a healthier weight and an overall healthier body.

Interestingly, studies have also shown that women who consume a lower-fat diet actually experience lower rates of breast cancer recurrence. In one study, this benefit was more pronounced among women with estrogen receptor-negative breast cancer when compared to those with estrogen receptor-positive disease. Of course, before making dramatic changes in your diet, it will be important to discuss these changes with your doctor. Many cancer centers have access to licensed nutritionists, so setting up a consultation may also be a great idea.

66. How do I cope with the fear of recurrence of triple negative breast cancer?

There are several ways you can address your fear. One is by talking to other people who have been where you are. Join a support group or take part in online chat rooms. Just expressing your feelings about this concern can alleviate some of the anxiety. You can also speak to a therapist or minister about these fears to get some emotional or spiritual support in handling them.

Once you've recovered from the effects of your treatment, work toward better health habits and a stronger body.

Another way is by taking steps to improve your overall health. Once you've recovered from the effects of your treatment, work toward better health habits and a stronger body. Improving your daily nutrition and exercise habits, quitting smoking (if you smoke), lowering your alcohol intake, and practicing relaxation techniques such as meditation are a few suggested strategies to help combat your fears.

Patient comment:

My main theory on coping is to try and stay busy. If I am in an online chat group and thoughts get too heavy I get offline and do something else, take a cancer break. If things become overwhelming in your mind or the fears start to creep in, then get busy, active, go out to lunch, see a show, call a funny friend, anything to distract your mind. I love laughter. Be around people who make you feel happy, laugh, and get out and enjoy something.

67. I have read that triple negative breast cancer can be quite aggressive. What happens if the treatment doesn't work? What if my breast cancer comes back?

Generally, if one treatment doesn't stop the cancer from growing, your medical team will switch to another—and if necessary, another, and another treatment. Like-wise, if cancer recurs in the breast itself, the team generally starts where it did with the original tumor—surgery, radiation, chemotherapy—but may choose a different method of any or all of these treatments. For instance, if your initial tumor was treated with lumpec-tomy and external radiation, your recurrence might require mastectomy and chemotherapy. If chemother-apy drugs were used in your initial treatment, a more aggressive regimen might be called for the second time around. It all depends on how your recurrence presents itself.

Although advanced or recurrent triple negative breast cancer can be treated successfully with the standard arsenal of treatments discussed in Part 8, there is no hiding the fact that with every recurrence or advance in stage, the stakes become higher. After repeated cycles of cancer treatment, you might need to recon-sider the goals of your treatment. Do you really want to continue going through chemotherapy and radia-tion with all the physical and emotional strains they place on you and your family in the hope of finally killing the cancer? Or would you prefer to switch to **palliative care**, care to relieve the symptoms of cancer and to keep the best quality of life for as long as possi-ble? There are arguments to be made for both approaches, which will be discussed later in the course of this book.

Palliative care

Care to relieve the symptoms of cancer and to keep the best quality of life for as long as possible without seeking to cure the cancer.

PART SEVEN

Behavior and Recurrence Patterns of Triple Negative Breast Cancer

I've just completed my treatment for early-stage, node-positive triple negative breast cancer. What are my risks for breast cancer recurrence?

If my breast cancer were to return, where would it most likely recur?

After completing my treatments for early-stage triple negative breast cancer, what symptoms should I report to my doctor?

More . . .

68. I've just completed my treatment for early-stage, node–positive triple negative breast cancer. What are my risks for breast cancer recurrence?

For women with triple negative breast cancer, the highest risk of recurrence is in the first few years after diagnosis, with the first 2 to 3 years being the period of highest risk. Unlike some other types of breast cancer, triple negative breast cancer rarely recurs after the 5-year mark. So, even more so than with other types of breast cancer, the 5-year mark is a very important milestone.

Your specific risk of breast cancer recurrence depends on several factors, including the size of the cancer in your breast, the number of positive lymph nodes, and the treatment you received. Your doctor will be able to give you an estimate of your risk of recurrence.

69. If my breast cancer were to return, where would it most likely recur?

In general, the most common places for breast cancer to recur are in the local area (i.e., breast, chest wall, lymph nodes), lung, liver, and bone. In comparison to other types of breast cancer, triple negative breast cancer is slightly more likely to recur in lung and slightly less likely to recur in bone. The brain is also a potential place for breast cancer to recur, although not often as the first site of cancer recurrence. At each visit with your doctor and/or nurse, you will be asked about any symptoms that might be concerning for recurrence of your cancer, and you will have a physical examination.

70. After completing my treatments for early-stage triple negative breast cancer, what symptoms should I report to my doctor?

At each visit, your doctor will inquire about symptoms that might be related to breast cancer recurrence. He or she will also discuss with you the symptoms that you should report if you develop them between visits. These symptoms include:

- New headaches, especially if they are severe and/or associated with nausea or vomiting
- Visual changes
- Weakness/numbness
- Problems with balance or coordination
- Difficulty breathing
- A cough that doesn't go away, especially if you did not recently have a cold
- Coughing up blood
- Chest pain
- Abdominal swelling
- Jaundice (yellow skin and eyes)
- Pain in the right upper part of your abdomen, just below the ribs (where your liver is located)
- Bone pains, especially in your back, hips, or ribs, and especially if they last for more than 2 to 3 weeks and have no other explanation (Fortunately, pain in the small joints, such as the elbows, fingers, knees, and ankles, is almost never related to breast cancer.)
- A new breast lump
- Bumps (could be skin-colored or red) on the skin of your breast or on the skin over your chest if you have had a mastectomy (or on the skin surface of your reconstructed breast if you have had a reconstruction)
- Red rash over the skin of your breast or on the skin over your chest if you have had a mastectomy (or on

the skin surface of your reconstructed breast if you have had a reconstruction)
- Swelling of lymph nodes, especially those under your arms, or above and below your collarbone

If you are not sure about a symptom, don't hesitate to call your doctor to talk. Many patients are hesitant to call their doctor between clinic visits because they are worried that they are "bothering" their doctor. But your doctor would much rather you call than worry and be anxious about your symptoms in silence! Often, by asking just a few questions, your doctor/nurse may be able to reassure you that your symptoms are not worrisome for cancer. Occasionally, your symptoms might be worrisome enough to prompt an in-person clinic visit and/or additional tests. Fortunately, most of the time, the tests come back negative.

71. If my doctor is concerned that my breast cancer has returned, what tests might he or she order?

If your doctor is concerned that your breast cancer has returned, he or she may recommend the following tests, depending on your symptoms and the level of concern:

- *Physical examination.* Elements of this exam will include listening to your lungs, feeling your liver, checking for breast lumps and skin changes, feeling your lymph nodes, performing a neurologic exam, etc.
- *Blood tests.* These tests will check your liver function, alkaline phosphatase level, calcium level, and often tumor markers.
- *Scans.* In addition to a CT scan of your chest and abdomen, and a bone scan, positron emission

tomography (PET) scans are sometimes done to help further characterize any abnormalities that might have shown up on a CT or bone scan. PET scans are not always necessary. Your doctor will discuss whether a PET scan is needed for you. If there is a concern for cancer in the brain, a CT scan or MRI of the brain might also be ordered.

- *Breast imaging.* Mammograms, ultrasounds, and/or breast MRIs are not always necessary. Their use depends on the symptoms you have when you see your doctor. Your doctor will discuss this with you.
- *Biopsy.* If the preceding tests reveal a suspicious area, your doctor may recommend a biopsy to determine whether the suspicious area is cancer (or not!) and to determine if it is a recurrence of your triple negative breast cancer or a new process altogether. The type of biopsy will depend on the area of suspicion. Biopsies can vary from a simple office procedure (e.g., a skin biopsy), to a biopsy through the radiology department (e.g., a liver biopsy), to a biopsy that requires an operation (e.g., some [but not all] lung biopsies). If you do need a biopsy, your doctor will discuss the specifics with you before the procedure.

Many patients find that waiting for tests to be scheduled and then waiting for the tests to come back can be a very stressful and frightening time. As you plan ahead, you may find it helpful to have a support person with you when you report for your tests and when you receive the results.

Talk to your doctor in advance about when to expect results and whether you will receive results by telephone or in person. If you are going to be receiving results by telephone, think in advance about whether you want your doctor to contact you at work or only at home. Doctors generally prefer not to leave such important test results on your voicemail or on an answering machine, so providing good times to call can be helpful. Many doctors also prefer to give results only in person, even if the news is good.

While you are waiting for your test results to come back, it is natural to jump to the "worst-case scenario." Fortunately, results of tests often come back negative, and your doctor will be able to reassure you that your symptoms are not related to a recurrence of cancer. At the same time, if you do have worrisome symptoms, it is important that you inform your doctor so that you can be evaluated promptly.

Fortunately, results of tests often come back negative, and your doctor will be able to reassure you that your symptoms are not related to a recurrence of cancer.

As you wait, it is also natural to want to start treatment as soon as possible. It is important that you have the proper tests, that you have a biopsy if recommended, and that the diagnosis of breast cancer is confirmed before starting treatment. Except under unusual circumstances, waiting a few weeks will not change how well you respond to treatment.

In the long run, having all of this information is critical in selecting the best treatment plan for you because the treatment of cancer depends largely on the type of cancer, your organ function, and other medical problems. Gathering all this information carefully and accurately can take time.

PART EIGHT

Management of Advanced Triple Negative Breast Cancer

My doctor has just informed me that my triple negative breast cancer is now "metastatic." What does this mean?

What treatment options are available to treat metastatic triple negative breast cancer?

My doctor has recommended chemotherapy. What choices are available?

More . . .

72. My doctor has just informed me that my triple negative breast cancer is now "metastatic." What does this mean?

Breast cancer can potentially recur in the breast (local recurrence) or in distant organs, such as the lung, liver, bone, or brain (distant recurrence). Occasionally, patients with a local recurrence can still be cured of their breast cancer. For example, a woman who had a lumpectomy and radiation in 2004, and then developed a new lump in her same breast in 2010, could have a mastectomy and potentially never be bothered by her breast cancer again. In contrast, when cancer spreads to distant organs, such as the lung or liver, it is considered stage 4 ("metastatic") and, for the most part, is no longer curable. The goal of care is no longer cure. Instead, the goal of care is disease control in an attempt to maximize survival time while maintaining quality of life.

Metastatic breast cancer is a serious diagnosis. Like many women facing this illness for the first time, you may experience shock, anger, sadness, grief, anxiety, regret, guilt, and fear. Please know that you are not alone and that what you are feeling is normal. Express your concerns with your doctor or nurse, and let him or her know if you feel you need additional support beyond that provided by your friends and family. Often, talking with a social worker or therapist experienced in the care of patients with cancer can be very helpful in sorting out all the emotions you may be feeling.

Although metastatic breast cancer is generally not curable, it can be treatable. In many patients, treatment can extend survival and improve symptoms. In practical terms, what this means is that you now have a chronic illness, one that will require ongoing treatment to be kept under control. When you were diagnosed with early-stage breast cancer, your doctor might have recommended a defined course of chemotherapy treatment (for example, four rounds of adriamycin and cyclophosphamide [AC]), after which you would hopefully be "done" with treatment. In patients with metastatic breast cancer, even if the chemotherapy is able to stabilize or shrink the tumors, without continued therapy, they would likely grow back, so treatments are continued as long as they are working and you do not have too many side effects. Your doctor may still be able to give you breaks from treatment ("chemotherapy holidays") from time to time, both to let you recover from side effects and to allow you to go on vacations or celebrate special events; however, it is true that by and large, you will remain on some sort of treatment to hopefully keep your cancer under control.

73. What treatment options are available to treat metastatic triple negative breast cancer?

As discussed previously, the goals of treatment for metastatic breast cancer are to prolong survival and maintain quality of life. Generally speaking, metastatic breast cancer cannot be cured. In addition, continued treatment is often necessary to keep the cancer under control. With this in mind, your oncologist will try to get as much mileage out of each treatment regimen as possible.

The goals of treatment for metastatic breast cancer are to prolong survival and maintain quality of life.

Treatments for metastatic cancer fall into two main categories: local treatments and systemic treatments.

Local treatments include surgery, radiation treatment, and other types of treatments. When patients are diagnosed with metastatic triple negative breast cancer, it is only rarely in a single spot. More commonly, there may be multiple tumors (sometimes called lesions) in the liver, lung, or other locations. Even if one or more of these lesions are removed surgically, it is usually impossible to remove all the lesions. For this reason, surgery (e.g., to remove parts of the liver or to remove the breast) is not commonly part of the treatment plan. Also for this reason, treatments like "chemo-embolization" or "radiofrequency ablation," which target specific spots in the body (e.g., the liver), are also not commonly used for metastatic triple negative breast cancer.

Radiation can be useful in a number of different situations. For example, if you have pain in a specific bone related to your cancer, a short course of radiation treatments can often rapidly relieve the pain. Radiation can also be used to control other areas of cancer, such as in the brain or spinal cord. There is a limit to how many times the same area of your body can receive radiation treatment; therefore, doctors will typically use radiation sparingly in order to have it available when it is really needed.

Systemic treatments include chemotherapy as well as newer treatments (sometimes called "targeted therapies"). Systemic treatments can be given either as pills or by IV. Because they are distributed by the bloodstream, they are able to kill cancer cells throughout your body, including in your lung, liver, bones, lymph nodes, skin, and breast. For this reason, systemic therapies are generally the most important part of your treatment plan.

74. My doctor has recommended chemotherapy. What choices are available?

There are many choices available for patients with metastatic triple negative breast cancer. Patients commonly ask what is the "best" treatment regimen. There is often not just one right answer, and the answer might be different from patient to patient.

If you received chemotherapy for your early-stage breast cancer (for example, adriamycin and cyclophosphamide [AC] or Taxotere and cyclophosphamide [TC]), you may remember losing your hair, being exhausted, and having other side effects, such as nausea, vomiting, or anemia. The types of chemotherapy doctors give for early-stage breast cancer are often different than the types of chemotherapy for metastatic breast cancer. This is because the chemotherapy treatments need to be tolerable over the long term so that you may receive them for many months (or longer) in a row. You might imagine that the "stronger" the chemotherapy (i.e., the more side effects), the more effective it might be, but this is actually not always true. While all chemotherapy treatments have some side effects, one of the goals of treatment is to find a chemotherapy drug (or drugs) that works against your cancer but still allows you to do the things you enjoy. Sometimes, the chemotherapy with fewer side effects can work better.

Some of the commonly used drugs include paclitaxel (Taxol), docetaxel (Taxotere), capecitabine (Xeloda), gemcitabine (Gemzar), vinorelbine (Navelbine), pegylated liposomal doxorubicin (Doxil), ixabepilone (Ixempra), cisplatin, and carboplatin. These drugs can be used one at a time or in combination with each other. Generally speaking, most oncologists will recommend that you receive chemotherapy drugs one at a time because there are usually fewer side effects this way. If your cancer is rapidly worsening or you have a lot of symptoms from your cancer, your doctor might recommend a combination of two (or sometimes more) drugs given together.

Some of the factors your doctor will look at when deciding which treatment to recommend are:

- What treatments you received before, when they were administered, and how you responded to them
- Your other health problems
- Your activity/energy level
- The potential side effects
- The likelihood of the treatment working
- The way the treatment is given (e.g., pills, IV infusions)
- How often you would need to come to the office for clinic visits
- Your goals and preferences
- Whether a clinical trial is available

Usually, the order in which you get different treatments is not as important as which treatments you receive over time. For example, if you start with Xeloda and then switch to Taxol once the Xeloda stops working, you may do just as well as if you had started with Taxol and then switched to Xeloda. For this reason, it is important to share with your doctor your goals, preferences, and priorities so that these can be taken into account in the decision-making process.

75. I want to be able to participate in the decision making about my treatment. How can I do this?

Treating metastatic breast cancer involves balancing potential benefits with potential side effects. It is important that you communicate your beliefs and values to your medical team so that everyone can be working for the same goals.

Many times, there can be several possible options, all of which are equally likely to be effective. Choosing between these options means weighing the potential side effects. For example, for some women, being able to take a chemotherapy pill and not having to report to the clinic for IV chemotherapy treatments would be an important advantage of one option over another. For some women, taking a treatment that doesn't cause hair loss may be very important. For others, the potential for fatigue might be an important consideration. Remember, for the most part, the amount of side effects from chemotherapy is not related to how well it will work. If one chemotherapy does not work, you may be able to try another treatment later on. By communicating your values and preferences to your doctor, you can help guide your care toward what is most important to you and what would maximize your quality of life.

Over time, your goals may change. At first, you may want to do everything possible to fight your cancer, even if it means dealing with side effects of chemotherapy and sacrificing some of your quality of life. But, there may come a time when your goals shift and you want to minimize the number of tests and procedures and to stop chemotherapy treatments (see Part 10). As you develop a relationship with your medical team, you will have conversations about your goals on a regular basis, and this will help your team to best achieve your goals.

76. Should I ask for a second opinion? If so, when is the best time?

Because breast cancer is unfortunately so common, most medical oncologists will have a great deal of experience taking care of women with metastatic disease. It is very likely that your oncologist will have taken care of many women with metastatic triple negative breast cancer over the years and will provide you with excellent care. But, it is also true that triple negative breast cancer can be difficult to treat; therefore, many women and their oncologists request a second opinion to help in the decision-making process. Also, there may be several treatment options to consider, and it can often be helpful to have another doctor weigh in to help you make a decision. Finally, you may want to consider participation in a clinical trial, which might require you to meet with a new doctor at a center where the clinical trial is available.

Treatment generally does not need to begin "right away." Exceptions are if you have an immediately life-threatening complication of cancer or evidence of severe problems with your organ function. Your doctor will let you know if this is the case. Most commonly, you could safely wait a few weeks to begin treatment. In that time, you can take the time to consider your options. Have discussions with your oncology team and with your friends and family. If you are interested in a second opinion, now is the time to seek one out.

In general, if you get a second opinion after you have already begun a treatment, the second opinion oncologist will recommend that you continue on your current treatment to see if it is working rather than recommending a switch of therapy. So, the most useful time to get a second opinion is *before* you start treatment, *or* at a time when your oncologist is considering a *switch* to a different treatment.

Remember that oncology is both an art and a science. Qualified oncologists can disagree about the best treatment. And there may be more than one right answer. You want to find an oncology team (doctor, nurses, staff, facility) that feels like a good fit for you. This might mean different things for different people, and that's okay. For some women, having access to an oncologist close to home offers peace of mind and convenience, both of which can improve quality of life. For other women, traveling a distance to a National Cancer Institute–designated cancer center to see a breast cancer specialist and/or to participate in a clinical trial feels like the right thing to do. Moreover, it is important that you feel you can express your thoughts and feelings, ask questions, report symptoms, and have what can sometimes be difficult conversations openly and honestly.

77. How will doctors determine if the chemotherapy is working?

After you begin chemotherapy, your doctor will examine you and check your blood tests (e.g., liver function tests) with each cycle of treatment. Usually, after two to three cycles of treatment, you will have a set of scans. The scans could include a CT scan, bone scan, ultrasound, PET scan, MRI scan, or some combination of these. Not all of the scans are always required; your doctor will discuss with you which scans are necessary at different time points.

Your doctor will use a combination of factors to determine whether the chemotherapy is working, including your symptoms, the size of tumors on your scans, whether new areas of cancer have appeared, and the results of your blood tests. Sometimes the answer is clear-cut, but other times, your doctor might recommend you continue treatment and have another set of tests after a few months to be sure.

If your oncologist concludes that your treatment is not working, he or she will stop the treatment you are taking and discuss the next steps with you.

On the other hand, if your tumors are either stable in size or shrinking, and if you are tolerating the treatment without too many side effects, you will continue on your current treatment. One concern that many women express is whether their treatment should be changed if the tumor does not shrink and instead remains the same size as before. Without treatment, tumors are likely to grow, so if the tumors are the same size, it can actually be an indication that the treatment *is* working. Although there are many different types of chemotherapy that can be effective, the list of possibilities is not endless, so it is very important not to stop treatments prematurely. Therefore, if your tumors are stable and you are tolerating your treatment, your doctor will generally recommend that you continue on your current treatment program. If your tumors have decreased in size, your doctor will also recommend that you continue on your current treatment.

So, what does "working" mean in relation to chemotherapy? Your oncologist will consider the chemotherapy to be working if it is at least keeping your cancer from getting worse and you are not having side effects that are too troublesome. As long as the treatment is working, you will continue on it in order to keep your cancer under control.

78. In addition to chemotherapy, my doctor has recommended I receive a drug to kill blood vessels that feed the tumor. Is this effective?

For tumors to grow, there needs to be enough blood supply to provide nutrients and oxygen. Many tumors produce factors that encourage new blood vessels to grow in order to increase their blood supply and allow the tumors to grow bigger. Scientists refer to this process as "angiogenesis." Several drugs have been developed that block this process of angiogenesis. The theory is that the drugs will cut off the tumor's blood supply and thereby starve the tumor of nutrients, leading to the cancer cells' death.

One drug that has been studied in breast cancer is called bevacizumab (Avastin). In one of the clinical trials, patients who received Avastin in combination with paclitaxel (Taxol) experienced a longer period of disease control compared to patients who received Taxol alone. In addition, there was a higher chance of tumor shrinkage or stabilization. However, patients who received Avastin did not live any longer than patients who did not receive Avastin. Of note, in this trial, the Taxol/Avastin combination was the first that chemotherapy patients received for their metastatic cancer. Based on results of this study, the FDA granted "accelerated approval" for the use of Avastin in metastatic breast cancer patients, meaning that the drug was approved, but the FDA wanted additional studies to be better understand Avastin's role in breast cancer. Since then, three large clinical trials have looked at adding Avastin to other types of chemotherapy to treat advanced breast cancer. These studies have generally shown the same conclusions: Adding Avastin lengthened the period of disease control. However, Avastin did not extend overall survival.

Because of these results, the Oncology Drugs Advisory Committee (ODAC) recommended against approval of Avastin for metastatic breast cancer. A final decision by the FDA is expected in the Fall of 2011. How the FDA decision will affect insurance coverage of Avastin is not yet clear. And, unfortunately, there are no tests available right now to predict which patients might benefit from Avastin and which will not.

135

Avastin has side effects, such as headaches, nosebleeds, high blood pressure, problems with kidney function, blood clots, and bleeding. There are other possible side effects as well. Avastin is not right for everyone. Your doctor will discuss with you whether Avastin might be an option for you.

79. I keep reading about PARP inhibitors to treat triple negative breast cancer. What are PARP inhibitors and why might they be effective to treat my cancer?

Both normal cells and cancer cells contain DNA. You can think of DNA like letters of an alphabet on a string. Depending on the order of the letters, different "words" are spelled, and when these words are put together, they create a message (a gene). In order for cells to function properly, the DNA creating a gene must be "spelled" correctly. If DNA becomes damaged, and if the damage is not repaired, cells will die.

Because of the importance of DNA, there are multiple pathways that your body uses to repair DNA damage. One of these pathways, called "base excision repair," depends on the functioning of the poly (ADP- ribose) polymerase (PARP) enzyme. PARP inhibitors are new drugs that block the function of the PARP enzyme. There are many PARP inhibitors in clinical trials, including olaparib, BSI-201, ABT888, and others. Some of these are given intravenously and others as a pill. By blocking DNA repair, the drugs are thought to kill tumor cells. By combining the PARP inhibitors with specific types of chemotherapy, the idea is to use the chemotherapy to cause DNA damage and then to use the PARP inhibitor to prevent cancer cells from recovering from this damage, thereby killing the cancer cell.

Early clinical trials of these drugs have been promising, especially in women who are BRCA 1 or 2 mutation carriers, and additional clinical trials are ongoing. However, none of the drugs have been approved by the FDA because it is not yet certain whether the drugs represent an improvement over existing treatments for triple negative breast cancer. You can talk to your doctor about whether there is a clinical trial that you might qualify for using one of these drugs. If you are interested in learning more about clinical trials, see Part 9.

80. What is the prognosis for patients with metastatic triple negative breast cancer?

It is impossible to predict exactly how long any individual patient has to live. Some of the factors that your doctor will look at are:

- How long ago was your original breast cancer diagnosed?
- What treatment have you previously received for your cancer?
- How long has it been since you last received treatment for your cancer?
- What is your functional status? That is, do you have a lot of energy and the ability to do all the things you did before, or are you in bed for much of the day because of symptoms from your cancer?
- What other health problems do you have?
- What organs are involved?
- Do you have any evidence of problems with liver, lung, or other organ function as a result of the cancer?
- What treatments are available to you, and what is their track record?
- Have you responded to previous treatments for your cancer?

Management of Advanced Triple Negative Breast Cancer

In considering the prognosis, the following questions can be helpful:

- On average, how long do patients survive from the diagnosis of metastatic disease?
- What is the chance of being alive in one year? Two years? Three years? Beyond?
- What is the worst-case scenario?
- What is the best-case scenario?

On average, if one looks at a group of many patients with metastatic triple negative breast cancer (i.e., all ages, different organs involved, some with other health problems, some very healthy except for the cancer, different treatments, etc.), most patients are alive 1 year after diagnosis. In the best-case scenario, some women are alive 2 or more years after diagnosis, and a few women survive for many years after diagnosis. Unfortunately, this also means that some women survive for less than 1 year. It can be difficult, if not impossible, to make accurate predictions when you are first diagnosed with metastatic breast cancer, especially since treatments, if they work, can potentially extend survival. However, these statistics are a big part of the motivation for oncologists and researchers to develop new and better treatments for triple negative breast cancer (see Part 9 on clinical trials).

Remember also that these survival statistics apply to a broad group of women with triple negative breast cancer. Your situation may be different. When you are ready, approach this subject with your oncologist. He or she will discuss these questions with you and individualize them to your specific situation.

PART NINE

Clinical Trials

My doctor has recommended I consider a clinical trial. What is a clinical trial?

What is the difference between a phase I, phase II, and phase III study?

I am worried about getting a "placebo." What is a placebo, and would I receive one as part of a clinical trial?

More . . .

81. My doctor has recommended I consider a clinical trial. What is a clinical trial?

There are many types of clinical trials. Some clinical trials evaluate the effect of new drugs. Other clinical trials evaluate the effect of other types of interventions—for example, changes in diet or exercise, counseling, or alternative therapies. Most clinical trials for breast cancer evaluate the effect of a new treatment on cancer (for example, a clinical trial to test whether the treatment decreases the size of your tumor(s) or how well it keeps your cancer under control). However, some clinical trials look at the effects of new treatments on well-being (for example, a clinical trial to test the effect of acupuncture on your energy level, or a clinical trial to see if writing about your cancer experiences helps you cope with cancer).

Before you participate in the trial, you will have a discussion with your oncologist about the pros and cons of study participation. You will have a chance to ask questions and to have your questions answered. If you do decide to participate, you will be asked to read and then sign a consent form that indicates your understanding of what is involved in the study and the potential risks and benefit. The consent form will also explain any tests, procedures, or treatments that are part of the study. If you decide to participate in a clinical trial, you will be monitored (with blood tests, physical examinations, scans, questionnaires, or other tests) at regular intervals as specified by the trial guidelines.

In general, clinical trials evaluating new drugs are conducted in different phases (see next question). The design of the study and the goals of the study are different depending on the phase.

It is important to note that all of the standard drugs used to treat metastatic breast cancer went through testing in clinical trials prior to their approval by the FDA. Clinical trials can provide a way for you to get access to new drugs before they are widely available. Many women also report that one of the most rewarding parts of participating in a clinical trial is the knowledge that they are contributing to progress in the fight against breast cancer and hopefully helping the next generation of women facing this diagnosis. At the same time, unfortunately, many potential new drugs that are tested in clinical trials for breast cancer fail to show a benefit. Thus, there is no guarantee that you would benefit personally from participating in a clinical trial.

82. What is the difference between a phase I, phase II, and phase III study?

Phase I studies are done to determine the dose of a new drug that can be given safely. In addition, phase I studies are done to find out what side effects occur with the new drug. Before a phase I study is started, the drug must be tested extensively in the lab and in animals. Typically, the starting dose in people is at a level where the researchers do not anticipate too many side effects. If the dose is tolerable, then the next group of patients will receive a higher dose of the drug. The process continues until a dose is identified that will be used in future clinical trials.

Many drugs are evaluated in phase I, but most do not make it to phase II, either because of the side effects or because there is no hint that the drug might be effective. If you are considering participation in a phase I trial, you will be making a very important contribution for future patients. There is a small chance you will be

Clinical Trials

directly helped by participation in a phase I trial; however, most patients do not directly benefit. Most of the time, participation in phase I trials is limited to patients with metastatic breast cancer who have already received at least one type of treatment for their breast cancer.

Once the dose for further testing has been identified in phase I, new studies will be started to get a better sense of whether the drug is effective and how patients tolerate the treatment. In general, phase II studies are designed to evaluate whether a new treatment is associated with tumor regression and/or stabilization. In addition, researchers want to better understand the side effects that might occur with the new treatment. Depending on the results of the phase II studies, researchers will decide whether to bring the treatment into phase III studies.

Phase II studies can either be "single-arm" studies, meaning that all participants receive the same treatment, or, they can be "randomized" studies, meaning that participants are assigned to one out of two or more possible treatment groups. Single-arm studies typically enroll between 30 and 50 patients (but sometimes more). Randomized phase II studies typically enroll between 80 and 150 patients. Compared to phase I studies, phase II studies often have fewer study visits and are usually somewhat less intensive in terms of how often participants need to see the doctor or have tests done.

Phase III studies typically will compare a standard treatment with a new treatment that showed promise in phase II trials. The purpose of a phase III study is to determine whether a new treatment offers a benefit to patients (in survival; prevention of cancer recurrence;

control of cancer, symptoms, or side effects; and/or quality of life) compared to existing standard treatment. In a phase III trial, patients are randomly assigned to one treatment or another. For example, a clinical trial might assign patients either to standard chemotherapy or to standard chemotherapy plus a new drug. Or, a clinical trial might assign patients either to the new drug alone or to standard chemotherapy. Neither you nor your doctor will be able to decide which treatment arm you are assigned to. Phase III studies typically include between several hundred and several thousand patients. Phase III trials are commonly conducted in patients with all stages of breast cancer, although the purpose of the study might differ according to whether the study is looking at new treatments for early-stage, locally advanced, or metastatic breast cancer. Unlike phase I trials, which are almost always limited to large cancer centers, phase III trials are often available both at large cancer centers and in community oncology settings.

Talk to your doctor about the pros and cons of study participation and the other options that are available to you.

83. I am worried about getting a "placebo." What is a placebo, and would I receive one as part of a clinical trial?

Some, but not all, clinical trials include a placebo. Phase I trials generally do not include placebos. Most phase II trials do not include a placebo. Placebos are somewhat more common in phase III clinical trials. A placebo could come as a pill, as an injection, or as an IV infusion. Placebos do not include any active ingredients. Your doctor will be able to explain to you whether a placebo is part of the clinical trial you are considering.

Talk to your doctor about the pros and cons of study participation and the other options that are available to you.

The purpose for including a placebo is so that researchers can better understand the side effects and effectiveness of a new treatment. For example, consider a clinical trial testing a new treatment for arthritis pain. You might notice from personal experience that arthritis pains tend to come and go on their own, with the weather, etc. Suppose researchers tested a new drug for arthritis and one-third of people reported relief of their symptoms. Was the improvement in symptoms related to the new drug, or would it have happened naturally without the drug? Similarly, what if one-third of people reported stomach upset with the new drug? How much of this was related to the new drug? By treating a comparison group of patients with a placebo, researchers can better tell what effects are directly related to the new drug.

In randomized clinical trials to treat breast cancer, the comparison group typically will receive standard care. For example, consider a clinical trial testing a new treatment for early-stage breast cancer. The "experimental" group might receive standard chemotherapy, such as adriamycin and cyclophosphamide (AC), together with a new pill that showed promising results in other studies. The comparison group might receive standard chemotherapy with AC together with a placebo pill. Note that *all* patients (even the patients who receive the placebo pill) receive standard chemotherapy, but half of patients might receive the standard chemotherapy plus the new drug. In general, randomized clinical trials are designed so that the comparison group receives a standard treatment that most oncologists would agree would be a reasonable choice for patients in their circumstance, even if they were not participating in a clinical trial. For clinical trials in breast cancer, patients almost never get just a placebo by itself.

84. What questions should I ask the doctor as I think about whether to participate in a clinical trial?

As you consider whether participating in a clinical trial is right for you, you may have the following questions:

- Why is this study being done?
- Why is this treatment being studied? Why do researchers think it might one day be a useful treatment for breast cancer?
- What do researchers hope to learn from this study?
- How many people will be included in the study?
- What does the study involve?
- How are the treatments given? How often?
- What are the possible side effects of the treatment?
- How often will I be evaluated, and with what tests?
- What are the potential risks?
- What are the potential benefits?
- What other options do I have?
- How long will I be in the study?
- What are the financial costs? Will my insurance company pay for part of this?
- How will my doctor determine whether the treatment is benefiting me?
- When will the results be known?
- Is there a plan to notify me of the study results when they are available?

85. If I decide to participate in a clinical trial, what might I anticipate?

If you decide to participate in a clinical trial, your doctor will go over the consent form with you in detail. Take the time to read the consent form and make sure any questions you have are answered. If you are ready, you will be asked to sign the form to indicate your understanding of the study, including the risks and potential benefits.

Once you have signed the consent form, you will begin what is called the screening process. You may have blood tests, scans, or other studies to determine whether you qualify for the trial. There is a small chance that the tests will show that you will not be able to participate. For example, if your liver function is abnormal, you might not be allowed to participate in the study because of concern that your body might not process the study drug properly. If the screening tests show that you do qualify for the study, you will then begin study treatment. Every clinical trial has a slightly different schedule of events—for example, how often you need to see the doctor, how often you receive your treatments, how often tests are done. Your medical team will discuss the schedule with you in advance so you can plan ahead.

Participation in clinical trials is *voluntary*. If at any point you change your mind, you can always decide to leave the study. Talk to your doctor if you are having second thoughts about participating in the study or if you are having side effects or other problems that make you concerned about continued study participation.

86. As part of the clinical trial, a research biopsy is requested. What is a research biopsy and what might it be used for?

More and more clinical trials ask for your permission to donate a sample of your tumor for research. For example, if you are participating in a study of pre-operative or neoadjuvant chemotherapy (chemotherapy given prior to breast surgery), you may be asked to undergo a biopsy of your tumor before and after the study treatment is given. Or, if you have metastatic breast cancer, you may be asked to undergo a biopsy of the tumor in lymph nodes, liver, skin, or another area before (and possibly after) study treatment is started.

Over the past few years, scientists have made enormous advances in our ability to study the genes and proteins in tumors. In the past, it might have taken an entire team of researchers several years to decode all the "letters" in the DNA of a breast cancer. Or, researchers might have been able to look at one protein (out of thousands) to see whether it is active in breast cancer. Now, scientists can look at thousands of genes at the same time. The hope is that with these more powerful tools, scientists will be able to better understand what makes a specific cancer behave the way it does, understand why treatments work against some tumors but not others, understand why some tumors spread but others don't, and understand how tumors become resistant to our current treatments. One day, this understanding may lead to important advances in the treatment of breast cancer.

Research biopsies do have risks associated with them. There is the potential for bleeding, pain, and infection. Depending on the area being biopsied, there is also the potential for other complications, such as damage to surrounding organs, although these complications are rare. If a biopsy is being requested as part of a clinical trial, your doctor will discuss the specifics with you in detail. Most of the time, neither you nor your doctor will get results of the research tests, and you will not personally benefit from the research biopsy. The hope is that results of the research will help other patients in the future.

Clinical Trials

87. If I decide a clinical trial is not right for me, will this be viewed negatively by my doctor?

After you discuss the potential risks and benefits of a clinical trial with your doctor and have had a chance to think things over, you might decide that participating in a clinical trial is not right for you. You should know that your doctor will not view this decision negatively. He or she will understand that a clinical trial is not right for everyone and will continue to take care of you. You will not be penalized in any way for saying no.

Talk to your doctor about the reasons you have decided not to participate. Are you uncomfortable with the idea of clinical trials in general? Were you worried about the potential side effects with the specific clinical trial you were offered? Do you have concerns about the number of study visits, the time commitment, or cost? Did you have concerns about being randomized or other concerns about the study design? Even if you decide not to participate in this clinical trial, there may be other trials for you in the future. Expressing the reasons for your decision may help your doctor determine whether there may be future trials that are right for you.

88. How do I find out about clinical trials that might be appropriate for me to consider?

Your doctor is often the best source of information. Ask about what studies are available through your doctor's office and also whether your doctor knows of other trials that might be right for you. You might also find it helpful to use the following strategies to seek out clinical trials:

1. Locate a comprehensive cancer center in your geographic region. The National Cancer Institute (NCI) recognizes cancer centers across the United States for their excellence. A total of 58 NCI-designated cancer centers provide care to patients. You can find the list at *http://cancercenters.cancer.gov/cancer_centers/cancer-centers-list.html*. Another good source is the National Comprehensive Cancer Network (NCCN) at *http://www.nccn.com/memberinstitution.aspx*. Contact the center to see if there are any clinical trials that might be right for you. Oftentimes, the cancer center will recommend you see one of the oncologists there for a consultation, and the availability of clinical trials will be part of the discussion.

2. Search the Internet. Both the NCI (*http://www.cancer.gov/clinicaltrials/finding/treatment-trial-guide*) and NCCN (*http://www.nccn.com/clinicaltrials.aspx*) maintain Web sites that will step you through the process of finding a clinical trial.

3. Search through the Web site ClinicalTrials.gov (*http://www.clinicaltrials.gov*). This site lists federally and privately supported clinical trials conducted in the United States and around the world. Select "Search for clinical trials" and enter key words in the search box (e.g., "triple negative breast cancer").

4. Call the National Cancer Institute at 1-800-4-CANCER.

5. Call the Coalition of Cancer Cooperative Groups (1-877-520-4457) or access the Web site at *http://www.cancertrialshelp.org*.

6. Call the NCCN Oncology Research Program at 215-690-0300.

7. Access the Centerwatch Web site at *http://www.centerwatch.com*.

PART TEN

Crossroads: Making Plans and End of Life

How and when will my doctor recommend that
I stop treatments altogether?

My doctor says it is time to move toward
palliative care. What does this mean?

What is an advance directive, and how can
I make sure my wishes are known?

More . . .

The goal of treatment of metastatic breast cancer is to sustain life while ensuring quality of life. You may reach a point in your breast cancer journey when treatments are no longer working and your doctor has no further treatments to offer. This discussion with your doctor will likely be the most difficult discussion you will ever experience and certainly the most difficult discussion your doctor has with his or her patients. Words may not adequately describe your emotions, which may include shock, frustration, helplessness, sadness, and/or anger. Although certainly not fair, you may be faced with this scenario. We hope that the contents of this special section may help to better prepare you and your family for this journey.

89. How and when will my doctor recommend that I stop treatments altogether?

There may come a time when you and your medical oncologist have a serious discussion about your treatment path. It may include a discussion about current treatments that are no longer working or the lack of additional treatment options available. Even if you would like to receive additional therapies, your doctor may indicate that your body has weakened to the point that additional chemotherapy is no longer safe for you. If this is the case, the benefits of additional therapies may be outweighed by the risks such that your quality of life is actually being compromised by your treatments. At this point, it may be time to shift your focus away from aggressive therapies toward preparing for end of life. There is probably no harder decision to make than this one.

In some cases, patients make the decision to halt therapy themselves, believing that focusing more on closure with family and friends and enjoying quality time with loved ones is more appealing than continuing aggressive therapies. It is important to know that there are no strict rules or specific guidelines to be followed when it comes to end-of-life decisions. You have to do what feels right to you. Some decide to continue treatment for as long as possible, while others choose to stop earlier. And, remember that the decision to stop therapy is not a permanent one and can be reversed if you wish. It is important that you not feel alone in this important decision-making process. Lean on your family, friends, and oncology team to help guide you through this difficult time, but remember to be true to yourself.

It is important to know that there are no strict rules or specific guidelines to be followed when it comes to end-of-life decisions. You have to do what feels right to you.

90. My doctor says it is time to move toward palliative care. What does this mean?

Palliative care is a philosophy of care that is intended to address your medical, physical, emotional, social, and spiritual needs. It is designed to optimize your quality of life. Though it was originally designed to help aid patients at the end of life, this approach to treatment and care is now available for patients in active treatment, too. In actuality, the management of incurable, metastatic triple negative breast cancer even while on therapy is palliative with the goal of controlling your disease in a way that you are minimally affected by your disease and your treatments. A key component of palliative care is ensuring that pain management is handled well. If pain management becomes problematic such that pain is not well controlled, your doctor may refer you to a palliative care specialist to help address this and many other end-of-life needs (i.e., emotional and spiritual health).

Crossroads: Making Plans and End of Life

91. I have had friends or family members with breast cancer who seemed to be diagnosed with metastatic disease for a longer period of time. Why has my disease moved so quickly, and why is my treatment list shorter?

There is likely not one answer to this complex question. Triple negative breast cancer is an aggressive type of breast cancer that is known to spread to sites such as the lung, liver, and brain. This is likely due to an inherent biology that drives both the rapid growth and the spread of this type of breast cancer. Not only is triple negative breast cancer a unique biology, but treatment options, as discussed previously, are mostly limited to chemotherapy. Luckily, newer biologic therapies (e.g., PARP inhibitors) are being developed and may turn out to be effective treatments for advanced triple negative breast cancer. Unlike hormone-sensitive or HER2-positive breast cancer, targeted treatments for triple negative breast cancer, including drugs like tamoxifen (which targets the estrogen receptor) or trastuzumab (which targets the HER2 receptor), are more limited. Thus, both the aggressive biology and more limited treatment options for patients with advanced triple negative breast cancer can compromise a patient's longevity when compared to other types of breast cancer. Try to remain hopeful. Scientists and doctors are conducting research every day to help better understand this disease and develop superior treatment options to help improve survival for patients with triple negative breast cancer.

92. My doctor says it is time to stop treatment and get hospice involved. What is hospice, and in what ways can I expect it to help me?

The mission of hospice is to improve the quality of life for individuals with health problems, both cancer and noncancer, and who are not expected to survive their disease. Hospice helps with many aspects of end-of-life care, including:

- Pain relief and other medical supportive care
- Emotional and spiritual support for you and your family
- Help with daily tasks such as bathing, dressing, and activities of daily living

Hospice services are usually provided at home (home hospice). Hospice can also be instrumental in helping reduce the financial expenses associated with end-of-life cancer care by obtaining prescription medications at cost; arranging for a hospital bed, wheelchair, and other medical supplies; as well as providing hospice nurses and home health aides to come to you on a routine basis. Most hospice agencies require that a 24-hour caregiver be with patients while providing 24-hour on-call services to these caregivers. A goal of hospice is to help ease the anxiety and stress caregivers may feel while caring for an ill loved one, while ensuring the patient's needs are being met. Some families are uncomfortable or unable to provide constant care of an ill loved one. Thus, an inpatient hospice facility may be the best option. Your doctor would help arrange such an admission to an inpatient hospice facility closest to your home. Hospice facilities have a 24/7 open-door policy of permitting visitors.

Hospice is different from visiting nurse (VNA) programs in several ways. The focus of hospice is on relief of symptoms, and support towards the end of life. The hospice program will often work with your doctor to set parameters for various medications. For example, you may be prescribed pain medications at a range of doses or medicines or treatments to relieve other symptoms. So, your hospice providers have more flexibility in adjusting your medicines and treatments compared to VNA. Although hospice cannot provide a nurse in your home 24 hours a day, you will have 24-hour on-call services to the hospice program in case problems come up. Many hospice programs include social workers and other trained individuals to help with all the many issues that worry you and your family, and some offer counseling to immediate family members as well.

Your doctor may also discuss with you "bridge-to-hospice" programs. These programs generally allow you to receive chemotherapy, radiation, or other treatments and offer a "bridge" between traditional VNA and full hospice services. Bridge programs can be helpful when you are still feeling generally well but need a little extra help. One advantage of bridge programs is that they are often run by the same agency as full hospice programs so you have a chance to develop longer term relationships with your home providers, and when the time comes, the transition to full hospice is easier.

Many insurance companies cover hospice care. If you are older than 65 years of age, you probably qualify for the Medicare hospice benefit. You may want to check with your insurance company if they have a relationship with a specific hospice care unit in your geographic region. For more information, call the Hospice Foundation of America at 1-800-854-3402.

93. What is an advance directive, and how can I make sure my wishes are known?

Advance directives are legal documents that allow you to state what type of medical care you want to receive if you are unable to make decisions or speak for yourself in the future. Although the specific laws and terminology for advance directives may vary from state to state, there are two basic types of advance directives: a living will and a healthcare proxy.

94. How do I get the correct forms to complete an advance directive?

You can obtain state-specific advance directive forms from your lawyer, your doctor, or your local hospital. If you were to be admitted to the hospital and didn't have one already prepared, you would be offered one to complete and sign, which would apply to you during that specific hospitalization.

The Partnership for Caring, a nonprofit organization whose mission is to improve end-of-life care, can also provide state-specific documents. They also provide information on other end-of-life issues and offer a national crisis and information hotline regarding this issue. For more information, please see the appendix.

95. What is a living will? Is this the same as a healthcare proxy?

A living will and a healthcare proxy are two different entities. A living will is a special document in which you give specific instructions regarding your health care, specifically focusing on measures to prolong your life. A living will can describe which medical interventions you would (or would not) approve of based on specific circumstances. As an example, if your heart were to stop, would you want CPR? If your breathing became labored, would you want to be placed on a ventilator?

As you make some of these very important and personal decisions, it may be helpful to differentiate between types of medical problems that might occur. If the medical problems are treatable and reversible, you may want all measures taken to resuscitate you and support you. However, if the medical problems are irreversible and there are no additional therapies available, you may not want to take extraordinary measures, such as resuscitation, to prolong your life. In that situation, some people may want to be explicit about their wishes and request to sign a "do not resuscitate," or "DNR" order. Making these decisions is very hard. Communicating with your family members may be emotionally challenging, but very important. It is really never too early to ensure that your wishes are known such that they can be carried out.

There are several limitations to a living will. Not all states recognize a living will. It is also impossible to imagine all of the potential circumstances that might occur in the future regarding your health. There may also be decisions that you simply haven't thought of or aren't ready to discuss and/or make decisions about. These types of problems may be solved by designating a healthcare proxy.

A healthcare proxy may also be referred to as a healthcare surrogate, a medical proxy, or a medical power of attorney. This person is authorized by you to make healthcare decisions on your behalf when you are not able to do so for yourself. He or she can decide which medical interventions will or will not be carried out, and which ones will be performed or withheld.

When you consider the person to serve as your health-care proxy, be sure to choose someone you trust and who will make decisions based on what you would want for yourself (not on what he or she wants for you). This person can be a family member or a friend. Talk with this person about what you would want to have done in the event such decisions are needed. It is especially important to discuss critical issues such as life-sustaining measures with artificial means (e.g., ventilation to help you breath) so your wishes are clearly known and understood. You can change your proxy at any time as well as change your decisions at any time.

Make sure your family and friends know who you have selected as your healthcare proxy. It is important for everyone to support this individual who is making decisions on your behalf. If you have completed a living will, share this with them as well. Inform your doctors and other members of your medical team what your wishes are, and give them copies of your signed advance directive documents. Each time you are admitted to the hospital, the staff should automatically ask you if you have these documents. If you bring them with you, they can become part of your medical record.

96. I am having difficulty approaching decisions about end of life with my family. How can I do this?

Having a discussion with your family about what you would want if you were unable to make decisions for yourself can be difficult for most people. Even if you have triple negative breast cancer that has not metasta-sized, you should be taking such steps, as no one knows what medical crisis may lie ahead. You may want to discuss your wishes with your family but may be worried that you will upset them. You may worry that while discussing these difficult issues, you may become upset. It is always best to have these discussions when you are feeling relatively well so you have a clear head and the energy to accurately communicate your wishes.

There are many ways to begin this discussion. You may start with something like, "I want to be sure that if I ever become ill, you will know what I want to have done." Sometimes family members don't agree with our decisions. This can make the discussion even that much more difficult. This is a good reason to have an advance directive so that your individual desires are documented.

97. I want my children to remember me. I also want to help them cope with my having to leave them. What can I do to help with both?

Young children often think they may have wished this on their mother. It is important for them to understand that they have not caused the cancer.

For very young children, it is important for them to understand that nothing they have done has caused this to happen. Young children often think they may have wished this on their mother. It is important for them to understand that they have not caused the cancer. They also need to understand that cancer is not contagious. Teens and preteens can feel significant anxiety and distress. Older children who are out on their own, even perhaps with their own families, will surely feel pain but are likely better equipped emotionally to handle the situation. For your children of any age, it is important to emphasize to them that they will be taken care of, no matter what happens.

As you consider ways to remain a part of your children's lives, consider getting cards for each of them—cards for every birthday through the age of 21, graduations, holidays, marriage, even their first child. Write a brief remembrance in each card to let them know you can still be "right there" instilling your values, your congratulations, your pride in their life as they grow up. Assign a family member or friend to be the keeper of your cards. Put the names and events on the outside of each card. Even go so far as to have the cards stored in a safety deposit box to ensure they are protected from fire, flood, etc. Select your family member or friend to be responsible for the timely distribution of your cards. Your children will sense your presence at the time of each milestone in their lives.

As you and your children face your illness, it is important to lean on not only your family and friends, but also your healthcare team. If your children are experiencing significant emotional distress, talk to your doctor about resources such as child psychologists or chaplains associated with his or her practice. It may even be helpful to bring your children in to meet your healthcare team so they know you are being well taken care of. This may ease some of their distress and anxiety about your illness, allowing you to spend more quality time together.

98. I am feeling distressed about my medical situation. How can I clear my head to think about what needs to be done?

At times, your illness may feel like it is too much for you to handle on your own. Sometimes it is advisable to seek the help of a social worker, chaplain, or counselor to help you work through your emotions. If already involved in hospice, let the staff know you are distressed. This is not the time to be stoic and hope that your feelings of anxiety will pass. You are in an extraordinary situation and it is perfectly normal to feel upset. You are encouraged to find ways to relieve your anxiety and reduce your stress. Here are some ways to do so:

1. Take a walk or exercise.
2. Journal your thoughts.
3. Meditate, pray, and perform relaxation techniques.
4. Talk through your feelings with a friend, counselor, or clergy.
5. Consider joining a support group for women facing metastatic breast cancer.
6. Join an online support group.
7. Listen to music that is soothing to you.
8. Create art or join an art therapy group.
9. Do yoga.
10. Spend time with close friends or family.

All of this is good for you, good for your family and friends, and good for the soul.

99. How do I decide how to spend my time if the doctor tells me it is limited? Do I work? Do I travel? How do I make these decisions?

Only you can answer these questions for yourself. We often go through our daily routine and forget to notice how precious life really is. It is not until we learn that our life is limited that we recognize its true value. Sit and talk about these decisions with your family and friends. You are not expected to maintain your old routine, particularly if you were feeling overloaded with responsibilities. You are in a unique position to make decisions based on what is important to you. If you enjoy doing certain things, this is your time to do them. It may be spending time with your family or taking a trip. This list will be unique to you. This is a time for you to express your thoughts and feelings openly and let people around you know what your concerns, wishes, and hopes are, especially for those you may be leaving behind. For many, this may be a very spiritual time. For others, it may be a time to rest with briefer visits from family and friends. Again, this is your time to decide what is best for you.

100. Where can I go to find more information?

The information in this book barely scratches the surface of what's available to triple negative breast cancer patients and their families. The accompanying appendix offers a selection of good resources to address many topics.

Crossroads: Making Plans and End of Life

Resources of Benefit to Breast Cancer Patients and Their Families

The American Cancer Society's Breast Cancer Network

American Cancer Society, National
800-ACS-2345
http://www.cancer.org/index.html

ASCO—American Society of Clinical Oncology

www.asco.org

BrainMetsBC.org

www.brainmetsbc.org

Breastcancer.org

www.breastcancer.org

Cancer Care, Inc.

www.cancercare.org
212-712-8080

Cancer Information Service of the National Cancer Institute

800-4-CANCER
www.cancer.gov

CancerNet-National Cancer Institute

www.cancernet.nci.nih.gov
900 Rockville Pike
Buidling #31, HSV2580, Room 10A046
Bethesda, MD 20892
1-800-422-6237

Cancer Research Institute

www.cancerresearch.org
1-800-99-CANCER

CenterWatch Clinical Trials Listing Service

www.centerwatch.com
581 Boylston Street, Suite 200
Boston, MA 02116
627-247-02116

Fertile Hope

www.fertilehope.org

Health Insurance Association of America

www.hiaa.org
202-824-1600
555 13th Street NW, Suite 600
Washington, DC 20004-1109

Institute of Certified Financial Planners

www.icfp.org
1-800-282-7526

The Johns Hopkins Avon Foundation Breast Center

http://www.hopkinsbreastcenter.org

Komen for the Cure

National Helpline 800-IM-AWARE
http://www.breastcancerinfo.com

Living Beyond Breast Cancer

www.lbbc.org
610-645-4567

Memorial Sloan-Kettering Cancer Center

http://www.mskcc.org/mskcc/html/11570.cfm

Metastatic Breast Cancer Network

www.nbcnetwork.org

Mothers Supporting Daughters with Breast Cancer (MSDBC)

410-788-1982
Email: *msdbc@dmv.com*
http://www.mothersdaughters.org

National Breast Cancer Coalition

www.natlbcc
800-622-2838

National Cancer Institute

www.nci.hih.gov
Public Office of Information
Building 31, Room 10A31
31 Center Drive, MSC 2580
Bethesda, MD 20892-2580
301-435-3848

National Center for Complementary and Alternative Medicine

nccam.nih.gov
888-644-6226

National Comprehensive Cancer Network

www.nccn.org
888-909-NCCN

National Consortium of Breast Centers

P.O. Box 1334, Warsaw, IN 46581-1334
Voice 574-267-8058 Fax 574-267-8268
http://www.breastcare.org/ or *http://www.ncbcinc.org/*

National Institutes of Health

www.clinicaltrials.gov

National Lymphedema Network

www.lymphnet.org
800-541-3259

NCCN-National Comprehensive Cancer Network

http://www.nccn.org

Partnership for Caring

800-989-9455
www.partnership forcaring.org/Advance/index.html

People Living with Cancer

www.plwc.org

Society of Surgical Oncology

www.surgonc.org

TNBC Foundation

www.tnbcfoundation.org

Y-Me National Breast Cancer Organization

800-221-2141 (24 hour national hotline)
800-221-2141 (24 hour hotline in Spanish)
Email: *info@y-me.org*
http://www.y-me.org

Young Survival Coalition

155 6th Avenue, 10th Floor, New York, NY 10013
212-206-6610
Email: *info@youngsurvival.org*
http://www.youngsurvival.org

Where can I get help with financial or legal concerns?

Accompanying any serious illness are questions and concerns related to expenses incurred as a result of treatment, health insurance questions that can be overwhelming to try to understand or resolve alone, and sometimes even legal questions related to employment or financial matters. Below is a list of national resources to aid you in addressing these types of concerns.

Cancer Care, Inc.

212-302-2400
800-813-HOPE
Email: *info@cancercare.org*
http://www.cancercare.org

Credit Counseling Centers of America (CCC America)

800-493-2222
http://www.cccamerica.org

Health Insurance Association of America

202-824-1600
800-879-4422
http://www.hiaa.org

Hill-Burton Free Care Program

800-638-0742
In MD call 800-492-0359
http://www.hrsa.dhhs.gov/osp/dfcr/

National Association of Hospital Hospitality Houses, Inc.

PO Box 18087
Asheville, NC 22814-0087
828-253-1188
800-542-9730
Email: helpinghomes@nahhh.org
http://www.nahhh.org

National Coalition for Cancer Survivorship (NCCS)

301-650-8868
877-NCSS-YES
Email: info@ccansearch.org
http://www.cansearch.org

Patient Advocate Foundation

757-873-6668
800-532-5274
Email: patient@pinn.net
http://www.patientadvocate.org

Social Security Administration

Office of Public Inquiries
800-772-1213
http://www.ssa.gov

Glossary

A

Acupuncture: A Chinese therapy involving the use of thin needles inserted into specific locations in the skin.

Acute lymphedema: A temporary condition that lasts less than 6 months in which the skin indents when touched and stays indented, but remains soft to the touch.

Adjuvant chemotherapy: Treatment given after surgery to increase the chance of a cure and to prevent the cancer from recurring.

Anti-angiogenic agents: An anti-cancer drugs that block blood vessel formation around and inside tumors.

Antiemetics: Anti-nausea medications.

Axillary lymph node dissection: Removal of lymph nodes in the armpit during the initial surgery; the nodes are then examined by a pathologist to determine if cancerous cells are present.

B

Benign: Not cancerous.

Bilateral breast magnetic resonance imaging (MRI): A non-invasive medical imaging technique used to visualize soft tissue structures, including the bilateral breasts.

Bilateral prophylactic mastectomies: Removal of noncancerous normal breast tissue to reduce the risk of another breast cancer in the future.

Bilateral prophylactic salpingo-oophorectomy (BSO): Removal of both ovaries and fallopian tubes to prevent a future ovarian cancer.

BRCA mutations: Mutations in either the *BRCA1 or 2* gene that leads to inherited breast cancer.

BRCA1: A tumor suppressor gene; certain mutations in this gene lead to an increased risk of breast and ovarian cancers.

BRCA2: A tumor suppressor gene; certain mutations in this gene lead to an increased risk of breast cancer, ovarian cancer, prostate cancer, and male breast cancer.

Breast-feeding: Breast-feeding is the feeding of an infant or young child with breast milk directly from female human breasts.

C

Cells: Basic elements of tissues; the appearance and composition of individual cells are unique to the tissue they compose.

Chemoprevention: Medicines prescribed to prevent cancers.

Chemotherapy: The use of chemical agents (drugs) to systemically treat cancer.

Chronic lymphedema: Lymphedema that lasts for longer than 6 months.

D

Delayed reconstruction: Breast reconstruction that is performed months after initial breast surgery.

Dosimetrist: Works with the oncologist and the radiation physicist to calculate the amount of radiation to be delivered.

E

Epithelial growth factor receptor (*EGFR*, also known as *HER1*): A receptor expressed on the surface of many cancer cells; EGFR is frequently over-expressed in triple negative breast cancer.

Estrogen: A female hormone related to child-bearing and the menstrual cycle.

External (beam) radiation therapy: The X-rays come from radioactive material outside the body and are directed at the breast by a machine.

F

Family tree: A diagram of a family's ancestry.

G

Gene mutation: An abnormality in genetic material that is either inherited or acquired; gene mutations can lead to cancer.

Genes: Sequences of DNA which comprise the genetic material of living organisms.

Guided imagery: A mind-body technique in which the patient visualizes and meditates upon images that encourage a positive immune response.

H

***HER2/neu* (Human Epidermal growth factor Receptor-2)**: A gene which is over-expressed in approximately 20% of breast cancers and can increase its aggressiveness.

Histologic grade: Describes how slow or fast the cancer is growing and progressing from stage to stage.

Hormonal therapy: Treatment that blocks the effects of hormones upon cancers that depend on hormones to grow (also referred to as endocrine therapy).

I

Immediate reconstruction: Breast reconstruction at the time of oncologic breast surgery (i.e., mastectomy).

Increased parity: Having many children.

Infertility specialist: A physician who helps women and/or couples achieve pregnancy.

L

Lactation suppressants: Medicines that stop breast milk production.

Lumpectomy: Only the tumor and a small section of normal breast tissue are removed from the breast, leaving the breast virtually intact.

Lymphedema: A condition in which lymph fluid collects in tissues following removal or damage to lymph nodes during surgery, causing the limb or area of the body affected to swell.

M

Malignant: Cancerous; growing rapidly and out of control.

Mastectomy: Surgical removal of the whole breast.

Meditation: A mental technique that clears the mind and relaxes the body through concentration.

Menarche: Start of menstruation.

Menopause: End of menstrual periods.

Metastasis or metastatic: The spread of cancer to other organs.

Modified radical mastectomy: The surgeon removes the breast, some lymph nodes under the arm, and the lining over the chest muscles.

Mutated: Altered.

N

Neoadjuvant chemotherapy: Adjuvant that is started before primary surgery.

Neutropenia: A condition of an abnormally low number of a particular type of white blood cell called a neutrophil. White blood cells (leukocytes) are the cells in the blood that play important roles in the body's immune system by fighting off infection.

O

Ovarian cancer: Cancer beginning in the ovaries, sometimes genetically related to breast cancer.

P

Palliative care: Care to relieve the symptoms of cancer and to keep the best quality of life for as long as possible without seeking to cure the cancer.

PARP inhibitors: An anti-cancer agents that block a tumor's ability to repair DNA damage.

Partial mastectomy: The surgeon removes the tumor, some of the normal breast tissue around it, and the lining over the chest muscles below the tumor.

Pathologic complete response: Disappearance of cancer cells in an organ (i.e., breast) following neoadjuvant chemotherapy.

Peripheral neuropathy: A tingling sensation in the fingers and toes that can become painful or interfere with daily function.

Perseverating: Uncontrollable repetition of a thought, despite the absence of a stimulus.

Premature ovarian failure: Early menopause.

Primary prevention: Any treatment method or lifestyle change that directly prevents cancer cells from forming, growing, or multiplying.

Progesterone: A female hormone involved in the menstrual cycle and child-bearing.

Prophylactic surgeries: Surgeries to reduce the risk of another breast cancer or a new ovarian cancer from developing.

R

Radiation nurse: Coordinates radiation therapy and patient care, helps patients learn about treatment, and assists in management of side effects.

Radiation oncologist: A cancer specialist who determines the amount of radiotherapy required.

Radiation physicist: Makes sure that the equipment is working properly and that the machine delivers the right dose of radiation.

Radiation therapist: Positions patients for radiation treatments and runs the equipment that delivers the radiation.

Radiation therapy (also called **Radiotherapy**): Use of high-energy X-rays to kill cancer cells and shrink tumors.

Radical mastectomy: Also called Halsted radical mastectomy; removal of both of the two chest muscles, as well as the breast and lymph nodes.

Radiotherapy (see radiation therapy): Use of high-energy X-rays to kill cancer cells and shrink tumors.

Receptors: Protein molecules that are embedded in the outside surface of a cell; when receptors are activated, cancer cells may be stimulated to grow.

Reconstructive surgery: The use of surgery to restore the form of the breast.

Reproductive endocrinologists: Doctors who help assess a patient's reproductive system and help the patient achieve a pregnancy.

S

Secondary prevention: Treatments or lifestyle changes that limit a person's exposure to cancer risk factors, but don't directly prevent the formation of cancer.

Segmental mastectomy: Removal of the tumor, some of the normal breast tissue around it, and the lining over the chest muscles below the tumor.

Sentinel node biopsy: The addition of dye during breast surgery to help locate the first lymph node attached to the cancerous zone; the node is removed to prevent spread of cancer and biopsied to determine whether cancerous cells are present.

Simulation: A practice treatment that allows the radiation oncology team to determine exactly where they want the radioactive beams to be applied.

Situational depression or anxiety: Feelings of depression or anxiety that are prompted by a specific life event or situation.

Stage: A numerical determination of how far the cancer has progressed.

Supportive care: Treatments devoted specifically to symptoms related to cancer.

T

Tamoxifen: A drug used to treat breast cancers that express the estrogen and/or progesterone receptors, called a selective estrogen receptor modulator (SERM).

Targeted therapy: Treatment that targets specific molecules involved in carcinogenesis or tumor growth.

Telangiectasias: Small red areas appear on the skin, caused by dilation in blood vessels of the skin.

Total (simple) mastectomy: The surgeon removes the whole breast, but does not remove lymph nodes.

TP53: A tumor suppressor gene; when abnormal cells can grow uncontrollably and form tumors.

Trastuzumab (Herceptin): An anticancer drug that targets breast cancers that express the HER2 protein.

Triple negative breast cancer: Breast cancers that lack expression of the estrogen receptor, progesterone receptor, and HER2 protein.

Tumor: A mass or lump of extra tissue; a tumor can be benign or malignant.

U

Undifferentiated: Cells that are not specialized and are somewhat immature.

Index

Index

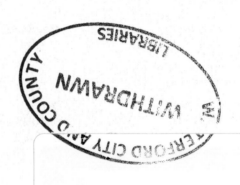